# Rollercoaster

# Rollercoaster:
## *a cancer journey*
re-inventing myself after diagnosis

## *by*
## Wayne Tefs

TURNSTONE PRESS

Turnstone Press
607-100 Arthur Street
Artspace Building
Winnipeg, MB
R3B 1H3 Canada
www.TurnstonePress.com

Turnstone Press gratefully acknowledges the assistance of The Canada Council for the Arts, the Manitoba Arts Council, the Government of Canada through the Book Publishing Industry Development Program and the Government of Manitoba through the Department of Culture, Heritage and Tourism, Arts Branch for our publishing activities.

The Canada Council | Le Conseil des Arts
for the Arts | du Canada

Canadä

Cover design: Tétro Design
Interior design: Sharon Caseburg
Printed and bound in Canada by Friesens for Turnstone Press.

**National Library of Canada Cataloguing in Publication Data**

Tefs, Wayne, 1947-
  Rollercoaster

  ISBN 0-88801-271-3

  1. Tefs, Wayne, 1947-  2. Cancer—Patients—Canada—Biography.
I. Title

RC265.6.T43A3  2002     362.1'96994'0092     C2002-910055-0

*for Marty, Edmond, Ken, and Ralph,*
*who have helped me on the cancer journey;*
*and for Kristen and Andrew,*
*who see me through each day*

# Contents

# Acknowledgements

Several of the photographs in the text are taken from sources. The photo on page 50 is reproduced with permission of Shering Corporation. All rights reserved. The photo on page 67 is reproduced with permission of the CARPA bulletin. I could not locate to seek permission, but would like to thank in any case both the meditation group for the photo on page 43 and the NCSG for the photo on page 64. I would like to thank the staff at Turnstone Press for their support and encouragement in bringing this book to press, especially Pat Sanders, judicious editor; Jeri Kostyra at Cancer Care Manitoba for the books and facts; Doctor Eugene Woltering of Louisiana State University, who kindly sent me useful materials about carcinoid studies; Monica Warner for her helpful notes on diet; Jeff Solylo for the photo on page 57; *Rays of Hope*, where the chapter "Radioactive Man" first appeared in a different form; Doctor Reg Friesen, an old pal who listened; Tristan and Liisa for their ongoing concern and hospitality; the Willow Island Gang for their good cheer; my former students who are now physicians, who have encouraged me to believe I am not alone; and all the nurses, physicians, pharmacists, and hospital staff who have sustained me along the way.

*Illness is one of the things which a man should resist on principle from the outset.*
—Edward Bulwer-Lytton

# Rollercoaster

# Prologue

*I have learned never to underestimate the capacity of the human mind and body to regenerate—even when the prospects seem most wretched.*

—Norman Cousins

I began writing this book as therapy for myself. After a number of years of living with cancer—at times not as successfully as either my wife or I would have wished—it seemed that putting down on paper some of my reactions to and thoughts about this experience might have a positive effect on how I was dealing with the disease. I hoped when I initially put pen to paper, in other words, to understand a little better what had happened to me over the years of anger, examinations, consultations, anxieties, therapies, treatments, emotional outbursts, and despondent periods that followed diagnosis. Perhaps, it seemed, such an understanding might lead to more effective methods of coping with cancer, more balanced daily living, more positive relations with my family, and even somewhat better health (I'm an optimist).

One of the subtitles of this book is *a cancer journey*. That is because what happens to us after diagnosis is similar to travel.

You will recall Marcel Proust's quip that real voyages of discovery are less about seeing new places than about seeing with new eyes. The cancer journey can be likened to travel, where we set off to discover things in the outside world, but come to recognize that discoveries at least as significant are unfolding inside our minds, spirits, and souls. Going on this journey takes us to places in our hearts we might otherwise not explore, but it also opens us to parts of ourselves that might otherwise remain hidden. Though we do not voluntarily set out on the cancer journey, it, too, involves voyaging into the zone of the imagination, where we confront unknowns within ourselves and then perform imaginative feats—among other kinds of acts—that lead us to redefine ourselves. In short, we undertake a parallel journey, matching physical actions with metaphysical questioning and spiritual quest.

I've also subtitled what I've written here "re-inventing myself after diagnosis." This phrase reminds me that we have two immediate reactions to learning we have cancer. The first is to think, *oh, my god, cancer, I'm going to die.* This is the initial response of shock, which is accompanied by anxiety attacks, and anyone who is diagnosed experiences its simple and direct terror. Hard on that response follows a second reaction, more complicated but just as intense: we flutter around, telephoning friends and relatives, and eventually our physicians. We need to vent our anxiety; we need comforting; we need commiseration. Understandably, we want to know the extent of our illness and the best and quickest ways to address it. What has worked for others—surgery, lecithin, Mayo Clinic? During this response period our reactions border on desperation; we don't sleep well and we have difficulty focussing on day-to-day tasks; we also think some things— again understandably—that seem to me quite wrong-headed, things that taken together I call the "toothache reaction to cancer."

Let me explain. When we have an infected tooth, we visit our dentist. He or she examines our mouth, takes X-ray pictures, studies them, and then explains to us what needs to be done to relieve us of the pain. We are suffering, so we think, *get the damn thing out of there!* The dentist employs one or the other techniques of "freezing" our mouth; she performs an extraction. There's some temporary pain to be endured, and then a little more as the freezing comes out. But in several hours, a few days at most, the pain—and its cause—is gone. We're relieved: the problem has been eliminated. Whoopee!

We adopt this attitude to other afflictions we have to endure: intestinal attacks, bee stings, thorns in the flesh, and so on. There's pain—remove it and let me get on with things. So when we are diagnosed with cancer, we would like to believe that a similar course will unfold. That is, that physicians can zero in on the area of our distress, then surgically remove the offending tissue, and leave us in a short period of time to resume our life much as we had been living it before diagnosis. Never skipping a beat.

But serious disease, certainly terminal cancer, does not work the same way as a rotten tooth. Disease or affliction or ailment is a sign that our overall organism, our body, our person is malfunctioning. Not one small and replaceable part, like a tooth, but the whole organism. And to address this malfunctioning in a way that truly speaks to it, we have to address what has been happening within our organism as a whole, within our self as a whole. For anyone diagnosed with a serious illness, understanding what is involved here is difficult: we do not want to admit that things in the big picture have gone awry for us, that our lives have come off the rails. We want to believe that we'd been living fairly sensibly. If you asked most people who had been recently diagnosed with a serious disease how they were doing just before the diagnosis, they would probably say, *all right*. No one has an easy time with diagnosis. So for some who become patients, dealing with diagnosis in a meaningful way can be even more difficult because in the end it means reflecting on who we are, on how we came to be that way, and on what we need to do to change our unhappy circumstances. It means self-reflection: examining ingrained behaviours, routines, and attitudes; it means

5

being willing to change how we live; it means, to use the subtitle of this book, re-inventing ourselves—or re-inventing our self.

This can be stated another way. When someone is diagnosed with diabetes, their life as they had been living it to that point must change. Diabetes cannot be removed by a neat surgical excision. With diabetes, as with most serious disease, something has gone wrong with the whole human being: it's enduring an affliction that involves the entire organism. The person does not merely have diabetes; the person, so to speak, has become diabetes (we commonly say: *is* diabetic, recognizing in that tiny verb the person's real status). And in order to deal with the illness, the person must alter eating habits, change behaviour patterns, monitor the organism's daily reactions to stimuli, chart insulin consumption, consult with physicians, and so on. To correct the ailment, alternative ways of living must be sought: sleeping or resting more, devoting intervals to non-strenuous exercise, taking time for play and recreation, meditating, and the like. In brief, to deal effectively with diabetes, a person diagnosed with that ailment must re-invent the self.

Most if us do not really want to undertake this. It's not a simple matter of popping a few pills. Nor is it the replacing of a defective part, as it might be when the refrigerator goes on the fritz. What has gone awry requires healing, and *healing* raises fundamental issues about how we see ourselves and how we evaluate the health system: for example, do we equate biomedical interventions, such as drugs and surgery, with recovery—or do we believe that if you die at peace with a terminal illness that you have been healed? This is another way of saying that genuine healing involves more than bones and blood and damaged tissue.

Some time ago a friend of mine suffered a serious internal attack to one of his major organs. He was hospitalized for some days. When he could welcome visitors, I went to see him. He looked drawn and tired and totally done in by his ordeal. He had suffered a serious episode, one that might have killed him. We chatted. He told me he had been experiencing the pain that brought on the attack for several months. He worked at his job very hard. He travelled a lot. He was under a lot of stress. He drank. During a subsequent visit, when he had begun to regain strength, I spoke with him about his traumatic experience. "It was awful," he said. "You've been through something like this," he added. "What do you think is the most important thing to do now?" I suspected that like most people he was looking for a simple answer, such as, *stop eating fried foods*. For that reason I've developed a certain reticence in response to such requests, but this was a friend of long standing, so I put to him what I thought was the most important question he now had to ponder: "Do you think this experience will lead you to change the way you live?" I was contemplating things such as backing off a heavy workload, or not travelling as much. Gearing down his hectic life. So I was thinking that what he faced was a re-assessment of certain behaviours; but it went farther than that: he was facing, too, a change in how he perceived himself. He looked at me in a quizzical way. "It's too early to tell," he responded. Several days later he was released from hospital. Within weeks he was back at his job, flying frequently, working long hours, as he had before—although he had altered his diet somewhat. For the most part, though, he continues to live much as he did before his traumatic experience, pushing his limits, bringing on stress.

Traumatic experiences, I believe, are messages, cries of help from our bodies. The import of the message our bodies are trying to give us is: CHANGE! It's my belief that we cannot go on living after such a traumatic moment in the same way as we were living beforehand. Maybe I'm mistaken about this. But we are not machines. If we are ailing, we cannot simply have a piece or part removed from our body and then expect to go on as we were before: healing the human being is not the same as fixing the refrigerator. Our organism in its largest sense is telling us to change. So in order not to provoke further trauma, we must transform some of our habits of life and our behaviour patterns, maybe the most important ones, adopting a new approach to living. That change involves a shift in how we view ourselves, as well as how we behave, an alteration in our persona. In short, we have to re-invent ourselves.

# Steamed Rice, Chicken Fingers, Broccoli

*To the destructive element submit yourself, and with the exertions of your hands and feet in the water make the deep, deep sea keep you up.*

—Joseph Conrad

On a blustery December afternoon in Winnipeg in 1994 I was standing in the living room of our house, looking out of the window, gripping a portable telephone in my hand. A physician was on the other end of the line, a gastrointestinal specialist. Doctor MF had an office downtown. His nurse/assistant was a brusque matron, whose attitude reflected, I came to appreciate, that of her employer. They were busy people, immensely competent professionals who communicated to me that they had no time to waste. I was that type myself. In late September they had performed a gastroscopy on me in one of their examining rooms. It had proved negative. Then in mid November, as a follow-up to the gastroscopy, Doctor MF had done a colonoscopy on me, searching for irregularities in my digestive tract and colon. That investigation had led to a follow-up liver biopsy, which Doctor MF had ordered done on me several days previous to his phone call in early December. He was, as I say, a man with gifted hands—and a diagnostic intelligence to match. He was also, perhaps, not the ideal person to be on the telephone with me at that moment, delivering the dark news he had to render. "Your liver biopsy has come back positive," he said. "You have cancer."

Since mid August I had been undergoing a set of routine examinations—ultrasound, barium swallow with X-ray, and so on, with an eye, I believed, to confirming a problem in the gall bladder. My symptoms were similar to those reported by friends and family who had suffered this malady. I was the right age for gallstones to have developed. So to hear *you have cancer* was both shocking and unexpected.

If you have never heard these words, it is quite impossible to fully comprehend their effect. I think immediately of an image from one of the Monty Python sketches, where a man strolling blithely along on a sunny day suddenly has a sixteen-ton anvil fall on him. I had lost my father to sudden death by heart attack two years earlier; had had a child born to me; had gone through a prolonged and painful marital breakup. These were all wrenching experiences that deflated me terribly, but really nothing to compare to those momentous words: *you have cancer.*

You know how it is when you have lost your wallet, or have become separated from your child in the mall: your heart races, blood rushes into your cheeks, you feel the top of your head lifting off your body. Perspiration, palpitations. Your hands go one way, your feet another, your mind yet another. Disorientation of the most profound kind. I have tried to reconstruct the moments that followed Doctor MF's words to me, but I cannot recall what I said to him. Perhaps, "Thank you." That seems pathetic and touching to me now, just the sort of thing a dutiful patient would say to assuage a doctor who should have known better than to drop that *cancer* bomb on an unsuspecting patient. Perhaps I asked, "Are you sure?" He was. No, I do not know what I said, but I do know I was looking for the umpteenth time at a fifty-foot ash tree in our front yard that had grown in such a way as to dangerously overhang our house; a tree that swayed in the wind and creaked and sometimes cracked—our neighbour had heard it too, and come over to warn me in case I had not heard it. I was looking at that tree and thinking, *we must get someone to cut that down before it comes crashing onto our heads.*

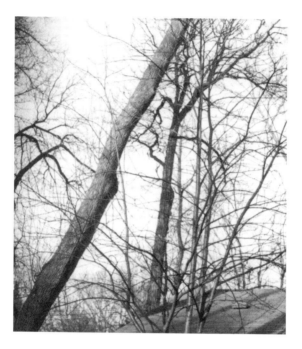

With the doctor's blunt declaration ringing in my skull, I put the phone down. I must have. To his credit, Doctor MF had told me one more thing: "The cancer you have is called carcinoid syndrome." But nothing else. The telephone went dead. I sat down—or perhaps paced nervously about. The house seemed much quieter than it had before that phone call. The hardwood floors made their little squeaking noises. The furnace was on, humming away and blowing hot air through the ducts. Some time passed before I did anything I can recall clearly. Possibly I wondered if I would live until

Christmas. I felt all right: strong, healthy. And acquaintances were always telling me that I was in great condition. Maybe I had a drink of Scotch to steady my nerves. Certainly I thought, *my son will grow up without a father,* and the image of my three-year-old boy made my insides go spongy.

I do know that for some time I was at a loss about what to do. Cancer. The worst possible thing that could happen to a person. Cancer. When I was a child in the fifties, there were two women in our neighbourhood who died of cancer, mothers of the friends I played street games with and shinny at the local rink. The other neighbourhood women, my own mother included, spoke about the affliction in whispers, much as they discussed teenage girls unfortunate enough to be "pg." *Cancer.* And with looks and sighs that almost made it seem as if the victims were to blame for having brought the disease upon themselves. They both suffered at length, these mothers of my schoolyard pals; they both died at early ages, and in doing so became both a cautionary tale for us, and one that made cancer seem as mysterious and lethal as the plague. Death. I was vibrating with an intense nervous energy: I felt the way you feel after drinking too much coffee—edgy, jumpy, unfocussed, and at the same time anxious. Over-anxious. Possibly I wanted to talk to someone—but who? K was at her classes at the Faculty of Law on a Friday afternoon. My sisters were both at work, and anyway, do you just call someone up— even a close sibling—and announce, "I've got cancer"? (It turns out you do—but more of that later.) My mother was alive but I knew I could not burden her; in fact, I had to protect her from this devastating news—the complete magnitude of which I did not myself comprehend at that moment. I did what most people do in the circumstances: I sat quietly and sipped at my Scotch, my mind at once completely blank and yet also awash with a thousand thoughts and images.

Of these latter the picture of myself lying on a hospital bed with intravenous attached was foremost. You know that ghastly anaesthetic smell of hospitals? The week previous I had just been through a biopsy-cum-CT scan, a frightening and painful experience, made all the more perturbing because I had gone through it alone and without much preliminary discussion with K; I'd been convinced the tests would come to nothing. I was active, healthy, and robust. I cycled, I lifted weights, I played on competitive sports teams. And now cancer. My expectation—and that of K—had been that I was suffering from a minor ailment. So I was in shock, yes.

I had been, especially in my twenties and thirties, an ambitious man. Raised in a mining town in the working class during the fifties, I had used education to improve my earning power and social status. I went to college; I graduated at the top of my class; I earned a PhD degree. I moved quickly along the career path I had charted for myself in my teens: college professor. Over the subsequent decade, the seventies, I taught at a number of universities. Students called me "Doctor Tefs." For a person of my modest background I had achieved quite a lot. I had been offered the position of Headmaster at the most interesting private school in the country. In addition, I wrote novels; they received critical praise and attained reasonable success in the marketplace. I was respected. I was planning on writing more books, on teaching creative writing, on . . . well, you know how it is. The prospect of cancer threatened all that.

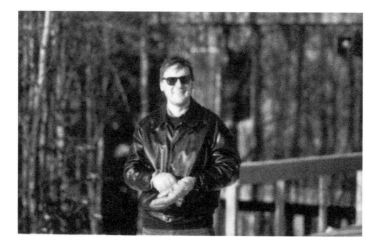

The surprising thing for me was not what I did when I put the phone down that day, but what I did not do. I did *not* scream and pull my hair; I did not fling myself on the floor and weep; I did not call anyone on the telephone and blurt out my terrible news. No gnashing of teeth; no cursing the gods; no sudden revelation as to the meaning of life. Maybe no one ever actually experiences those dramatic things; maybe they are only the stuff of the afternoon soaps and the tabloid press. Hand-wringing histrionics.

As the minutes, and then the hours, unfolded, I came to an unusual discovery, one that to this day causes me to marvel at the resilience of the human being: even when the worst thing you can conceive happening to you does happen to you, you go on. Life goes on. I had always imagined that in a moment like this I would collapse or undergo an instant conversion in my philosophy—like Saul on the road to Damascus—but instead I drank my glass of Scotch; I went to the bathroom and had a pee; I rummaged about in the kitchen as I waited for K to come home from her classes. I paced about. I kept coming back to the living-room window. A trick of the light and the triple-glazing reflected my own image back to me: big jaw, glasses, a shock of unruly brown hair. I put my fingers on the glass: it was chill to the touch. After a while I leaned my forehead on the cool glass and stood that way for some time, as if in a trance.

When I roused myself, I realized that the day was waning, that K would soon be returning home. Routine is what we humans live by, disaster or no, and I fell back on my routines; I started making preparations for supper: steamed rice, chicken fingers, broccoli.

-So, you're Wayne.

-And you're cancer. What else is there to say? I hate you. End of story.

-We don't really care. But you started, you—

-Look, I hate you. My guts knot up when I think of you. Yes. At the mere thought of you—*cancer*—bile and spit rise in my mouth. I taste the stink of you. My fists ball up, and veins in my temples stick out, throbbing with the pulse of blood, blood that you have contaminated. My heart leaps and I want to smash something!

-Poor baby.

-I jump from my chair, and I rage in a blind fury, punching the first thing that comes into range, the door of my studio. I smash it. It rockets open, bashing into the wall behind it. I scream: *Why me?* I scream: *Goddamn it, why me?*

-Yes, you would. *Me, me.* Essentially you're a big baby.

-Pain races through my fingers. My wrist throbs; I've jammed something there, muscles or tendons or whatever, they scream out—STOP! But I'm out of control; I strike again and again.

-Primitive anger, dear boy. A man going off the deep end. Male rage.

-I hate you, I want to kill you.

-This ranting makes you a cliché.

-I would pulverize you, reduce you to pulp and blood. Reduce you to a pile of shit.

-But you can't.

-I cannot and the rage is so great I kick the wall.

-You're a baby. But you insist on your fits. So, why are you here at all? Why bother to start talking?

-Not my idea. EB's idea, K's idea. "Look inside yourself, open up a dialogue with your cancer." Crap.

-Ditto from this side. We prefer to work silently from within, to grow secretly.

-You mean kill me.

-Dear boy. It's not personal.

-You eat up the good cells, you destroy healthy tissue, you reduce me to a pile of shit.

-Such bile and name-calling. There's no malice. Cancer simply is. You don't come knowing that?

-I come out of desperation. Out of fear and anger and desperation.

-At least that's honest.

-Piss off.

-*As you will.*

# Hot Dogs,
# Chips and Crackers, Cokes

*Everyone who is born holds dual citizenship, in the*
*kingdom of the well and in the kingdom of the sick.*
*Although we all prefer to use only the good passport,*
*sooner or later each of us is obliged, at least for a*
*spell, to identify ourselves as citizens of that other*
*place.*

—Susan Sontag

Throughout the summer of 1994 I had been experiencing
minor gastrointestinal attacks. The symptoms were fairly
common: upset stomach in the middle of the night, burp-
ing, "gas," a general uneasiness in the guts that led to brief
periods of sleeplessness between three and five AM, followed
by a morning of mild headache accompanied by queasiness
and discomfort. "Borborygmi" is the word I encountered for
these symptoms years later, a word that as a writer I immediately formed an attachment to, despite the fact I have no
taste for the symptoms themselves that borborygmi
describes.

A number of acquaintances surmised that I was experiencing acid reflux, a fairly common minor ailment that develops

in people of my age at the time of life when I was diagnosed, the mid/late forties. Perhaps gallstones, conjectured others.

When I thought about the symptoms I was enduring—and I did not at first give them much thought—they seemed to be occasioned by the eating of fatty foods, or the drinking of white wine. On a particularly memorable occasion, memorable for the severity of the pain I suffered, I had eaten barbecued salmon the evening before at a family gathering and consumed with the meal several glasses of wine. The following day, a Sunday, I spent most of the afternoon in minor discomfort: grainy headache, a rocky gut, restlessness, irritability, the symptoms commonly lumped together under "hangover." The usual remedy for gut upset, Tums, had not helped. The symptoms persisted. I felt like vomiting.

These were warning signs, I realize now, my body telling me something was amiss. I did not know this at the time, that our bodies tell us when things are going wrong, or that our general health is under duress. That we should stop doing the things we're doing—and immediately! We're not accustomed to listening to internal signals. In our culture we tend to think of our bodies as machines that can be driven along at pretty much whatever hectic pace we determine for them, flinging Tylenol and Tums into our throats when the body periodically speaks out with symptoms such as headache or gas. Television commercials for these remedies do not help: in fact, they cultivate this slapdash approach to health. Such commercials tell us, *just take a couple of Tums or Aspirin and your pain will vanish.* Until we have had a serious illness—or lived with someone who has—we do not register the multiple signals our bodies send out to us, warning us that we're in the downdraft of impending illness and that much more serious things may soon befall us. (I once read an interesting quip about this whole business: "Having a headache doesn't mean you're low on Tylenol.")

Probably a wiser person, a person more in tune with his whole being, would have heard his body speaking out much earlier than I did. When I reflect back now, I realize I'd been experiencing borborygmi for years, though not seriously enough to prompt me to ask questions about why I was "gassy," or to consider changing any of my consumption habits. (Give up cold beer and potato chips and pickled eggs at midnight—I think not!) Since then I have asked myself this question: would having been more in tune with my body—listening to its messages—have made any difference, prevented the contracting of cancer? There's no way to know, really. But I think so. Certainly when I listen to my hungover athletic pals complaining about their stomach twinges and intestinal afflictions, I overhear a version of my pre-diagnosis self, and I sense my locker-room mates should be complaining less about their gut aches and acting more positively to address their bodies' messages. Well, that's easy to say now.

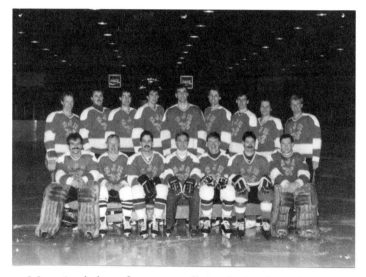

My pains led me first to a walk-in clinic where the attending physician informed me there was nothing she could do to help. "Go to Emergency," she told me. This was shocking advice. I'd expected some pat response—"Try Maalox"—or some such thing, and when I came out of the walk-in clinic it first dawned on me that something fairly serious was about to be revealed to me. I'd screwed up in a more than minor way.

I remember saying to K in a shaky voice, as we drove to the emergency ward of the nearest hospital, "I know what's wrong; I've got an ulcer. Shit." I was bent over in the passenger's seat of the car, nursing the ache in my gut and feeling sorry for myself and just a little resentful about the indignity of ulcers. I pictured myself unable to drink alcohol or enjoy certain foods: chili and pizza. Terrible limitations on my life, I imagined then.

If only, I've had occasion to think often since.

The physicians and nurses I encountered at the emergency ward were very kind. It took them some time to get me stable and to try various antidotes for the continuing pain I was experiencing in my abdomen. Finally they hit upon the "pink lady," a mixture of Maalox and the freezing agent xylocaine, that effectively numbed the aggravation in my gut so that I could rest easily for a period—and even sleep. Doze, anyway. Around midnight, rested and somewhat stronger, K and I stumbled out of the hospital, armed with a prescription for an intestinal corrective, ranitidine, and the sage advice that I should visit my family doctor immediately or run the risk of having an "attack" reoccur.

Coming out of the emergency ward that night, I recall looking at the sky. It was late August. A harvest moon shone brightly far overhead. A peculiar light coloured the horizon in

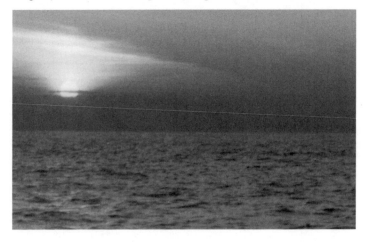

all directions, a rosy mixture of pink and purple, a boreal bruise. I recall saying something to K about it: raised in the country, she has an attachment to expansive, open spaces and the western sky at dusk. We stood looking at that livid sky for a few minutes, hand in hand, before we roused ourselves to the task before us: making an appointment with M, our family doctor.

The visit to M led to the gastrointestinal specialist, Doctor MF. At the time I was convinced I had developed gallstones, or at worst had an ulcer, and was expecting to hear from him that I would no longer be able to eat and drink the things I had grown used to consuming over thirty years of adult life characterized by blithe unconcern and willful indulgence— pizza, beer, burgers, fries, gravy, hot dogs, chips, crackers, Cokes, nachos, melts. What I thoughtlessly dumped into my body in those days causes me to wince now.

So I was surprised when Doctor MF performed a gastroscopy (uncomfortable—gagging, sweating, flatulence) on me in his office and informed me that nothing was amiss in my stomach. I asked, "No ulcer?" He responded, "No, you're okay there." If I'd been listening closely I'd have heard the ominous ring in that final word. Doctor MF was suspicious that something more serious than ulcer was going on in my guts. But I was too relieved—and no doubt too busy—to recognize that he was not relieved. He set me up for a colonoscopy at the hospital where he did these things and a week later performed that spectacularly uncomfortable procedure. "There's something high up in your lower intestine," he informed me when he took a brief break from worming his instrument up into my bowel, sweating considerably himself. "I can see it but I cannot biopsy it; I'm concerned about causing you more discomfort than I already have." He was right to be concerned: of the many diagnostic procedures I've undergone since, colonoscopy is not only the least dignified, it's also the most exquisitely painful. (A woman acquaintance told me, "I've had children both ways, and believe me, those pains are nothing compared to the colonoscopy I endured.")

21

On the same day as he performed the colonoscopy, Doctor MF had arranged for a radiation scan to be done on my intestines. A number of us undergoing the procedure drank two gigantic cups of barium (boy, did that settle our stomachs!) and then stood in the hospital corridor—*stood* so the barium could more easily make its way through our gastrointestinal tracts—and waited our turn for the radiation pictures. There was a young man standing beside me, maybe thirty years of age, a man with a thin blond beard and a pot belly. He wore what were once expensive training shoes, streaked with dirt and badly collapsed at the heels. He was pale and sweating. He told me he was there to confirm Crohn's disease. I remember feeling sorry for him, and cannot help but remark now on my own hubris: there I was waiting to be X-rayed and feeling pity for him; standing in that line-up, being tested for what would ultimately prove to be cancer, I nevertheless was incapable of recognizing that I was in at least as grave a predicament.

Well, we don't want to acknowledge these things, do we? Men of my generation and disposition will go a long distance out of our way to avoid acknowledging the bad things happening to us. On the one hand, it's a self-preservation instinct, a good thing; on the other, it's just willful blindness that can easily devolve into our own undoing.

It turned out that the radiation pictures revealed spots on my liver, confirmed by an ultrasound days later. These tests were followed by a liver biopsy. I was becoming quite familiar with the corridors of the Saint Boniface Hospital. I had not in my adult life been in any area of a hospital other than an emergency ward—for "stitches" to repair sports lacerations—so the chain of experiences I had undergone in a brief month-long period somewhat unnerved me: so many people in white coats, padding around in squeaky shoes, looking competent and busy and grave (that last observation concerned me). I was busy, too, I recognize now, denying what I must have realized, unconsciously at least, denying what was being communicated to me by all these visits: something perhaps deadly serious was wrong with me.

A liver biopsy is performed in accompaniment with a CT scan: using a lengthy syringe, the physician probes into the liver at places where tumours appear on the scan. In my case, the tumours (at least the ones the physician could gain easy access to) were small, so small that he had to repeatedly set and re-set his—it seemed—enormous biopsy needle. I had been given a local anaesthetic in my side, so the probing felt similar to that in the dentist's chair, remote but definitely uncomfortable: an abstracted pressure that from time to time would intensify suddenly and sharply, causing me to flinch and feel nauseous. You know that sickening trauma you experience when a nurse cannot quite locate the vein in the crook of your arm and has to keep poking about with the needle—sweating, nausea? Imagine that several times magnified as you lie on your back in the unfamiliar and frightening environs of the CT scanning room, breathing in the anaesthetics of the hospital, dreading the worst, and listening to the bleeping of the scanner, behind which ominous sound you can just hear the physician telling the nurses in a subdued and harried voice that he's having a great deal of difficulty procuring a biopsy sample.

For a CT scan to work, certain liquid dyes, "contrasts," the attendants call them, are run through your veins as you lie in the scanner. These have three side effects, none of which is pleasant: a metallic taste at the back of your mouth; hot flushing through the abdomen and groin; the urge to urinate. After an hour or so the sweat in my armpits and on my forehead had built up. The fretful responses of my mind matched those of my body, surpassing anxiety and bordering on hysteria.

The technician, the nurses, and the doctor performing the biopsy, a Doctor Q, conferred in whispers from time to time. Besides the concern in their voices, I heard the words "bruising" and "multiple." I had only a confused sense of what was happening to me. It was not going well. The room was large and, except for the scanning machine and one bench, empty; the scanning machine was a muted shade of brown; everyone was clad in white gowns and moved ethereally around my supine body. It seemed I had entered a ghostly other world where the attending sprites drifted about in squeaky shoes.

In my cancer journey I have had the good fortune to run into many fine physicians and nurses. On this particular occasion, a younger nurse sensed my discomfort as well as the fear that was wracking me. Allison, her name tag read. She did something unusual and something for which I am grateful to this day. About half an hour into the painful and numbing CT scan-cum-biopsy—numbing because you're required to hold your arms locked back over your head during a CT scan, one with a throbbing intravenous attached—Allison freed the fingers of one of my hands from the other and took it in hers.

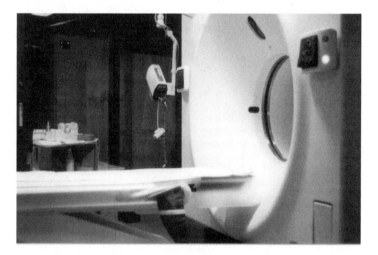

She held my hand and gently squeezed the fingers. Simply that: warm flesh and bone of one person gripping another. A wordless and comforting gesture that told me I was not—as I really had begun to expect—going to die right there in the scanning room. A gesture that told me I was not alone.

Her comforting gesture probably helped me relax, and, with the dose of local anaesthetic to ease the pain in my side, drop into a grainy and restive trance as we neared the conclusion of the procedure. By the time I reached the recovery room I was in considerable distress. I may have lost consciousness in between the CT scan area and Recovery. Perhaps I was given another mild sedative. I do not recall being wheeled from the one location to the other. But when I again became aware of my surroundings, I realized there were smells other than anaesthetic about, and nurses were here and there, one of them offering me something to drink. The man in the bed beside me grunted. When I shifted about to acknowledge him, he nodded and grunted again in that way I've since come to recognize as the universal signalling system of veterans of hospital procedures: it says, *don't feel any pressure to enter a conversation, but if you're willing to parley, I am too.*

In my own wordless way I must have let him know that I was open to talk.

He was Slavic, this man: I recognized in the way he spoke the accents of the sometime immigrant. Remember the way Steve Martin and Dan Aykroyd, those "wild and crazy guys," used to gabble on when doing that "American foxes" routine on the old *Saturday Night Live*? He must have known, this Slavic man, what I did not: that we were in the biopsy recovery area. He was eating something, consommé soup, perhaps, but he leapt immediately to the heart of the matter, saying to me, "Fifteen years ago the doctors told me I had five years to live." He pointed to his side. He was wearing a colostomy bag. "Fifteen years," he repeated, "they give me. I was scared then, but not so much now. It's not so bad," he went on. He stopped to slurp at his soup. "I quit work. I make Christmas dinner for my whole family, turkey, cabbage rolls, the whole works, lots of fun. They cut an entire section out of my guts. Not once, but twice. It's not so bad. You get used to it. Fifteen years, see, and they told me five." He settled back into his pillows, satisfied with his survival story and happy to have made his point to me.

I've thought of that man often since. I was too tired and too worn down to realize at the time the full import, much less the wisdom, of what he was telling me. Yet his simple but encouraging assessment, like Allison's simple human touch, was a gesture of both dignity and comfort, a way for me to see past the pain of the moment to something better just a little way down the road. People with terminal diseases often reveal this little genius: the capacity to look past their own pain and grief in an upbeat way that lifts your spirits too. Cancer patients can be remarkably positive. A radiologist I encountered once was contemplating switching specialties, just because, as he put it, "You people are so darn upbeat." On the whole, cancer patients are wiser than they were before the illness that has befallen them; more generous with hope, and more daring in their capacity to encourage you to hope, too; their optimism, transmitted in their eyes and in their voices, can help you begin the journey toward the new self that you are about to become.

"It's not so bad."

His off-hand comment seemed miles removed, psychologically speaking, from most other people's first response to *cancer*. But he was right.

-I won't ask, *why me?* Not today. But I will ask this: where did you come from?

-Do give over, dear boy. From inside your body.

-No. You are an alien thing, you're an intrusion from outside. An ugly parasite that attaches to an innocent host, an evil that attacks a good. A canker.

-Oh, my. Not true. Cancer is an inexorable fact. But neutral. See, we are you, the same as your nose is you, the same way each follicle of your hair is you.

-I will not accept that. You are a hateful sore, a scab dribbling pus.

-You want to call names? You don't want to talk? Fine. Let it be silence. Let us go back to working silently and secretly within.

-No. That is no good. Goddamn you, but that is no good any longer.

-What then?

-A better question: not where did you come from—but why did you come?

-We came because we could: we grew as a wart grows on the back of your hand.

-No, that's crap. Cancer comes to punish people. They've done something hurtful, a bad thing. So you came to punish me—for something I'd done wrong, for being bad, for betrayals or failures. That sort of thing.

-You still haven't got it. We do not arrive as retribution. We do not come to punish for moral failures—or any other kind of failure. We come because the time is ripe.

-I was ripe?

-Your body was.

-This is silly talk.

-Dear boy, stop railing for a moment and think about what happened in the year or so prior to the time you were diagnosed.

-OK. In that time span these things occurred: my father died; I left my job; I moved out of the house where my former wife and I had lived for years; then she moved out.

-That's quite a list, see.

-So you were waiting, waiting to move in on me, you mean?

-All that stress. You were drinking too. Not sleeping well.

-I became weak. That's what you're saying. I let myself weaken and you seized the moment and started to develop. Pounce!

-You want to turn this into a soap opera. OK. Have it your way. But it's worth saying again: cancer is not retribution for moral failure, or the dark harvest of not having "looked after yourself."

# Bandages
# and Tongue Depressors

*Reports of my death are greatly exaggerated.*
—Mark Twain

On the Monday following the Friday when Doctor MF told me, *You have cancer*, my family physician, M, called. Actually, it was the receptionist at M's office who called to tell me that I had an appointment with an oncologist (I had never heard the word before). His clinic, Doctor N's, was conducted, I was informed, in an office tower in the downtown area. On Tuesday, still reeling from the shock of having cancer, and no more knowledgeable about carcinoid syndrome than I had been on the previous Friday, I arrived at Doctor N's office. Or rather, at Doctor N's waiting room.

I was not familiar at that time with the outer waiting room (proceed to) inner waiting room routine, which is the standard procedure in the world of medical clinics today. It was hot and stuffy. It seems always to be overly warm and stifling in waiting rooms. I realized I should have brought a book to pass the time. There were magazines to flip through in the outer office, and other patients to study. Did they all have cancer? Many were accompanied by loved ones—

husbands, wives, mothers, daughters. Some held hands. I peeked at them over the top of my two-month-old sporting magazine: no one looked to be in critical condition, but everyone seemed tense, holding their breath. Everyone was talking in the subdued voices we all—except children and the mentally challenged—assume in waiting rooms at clinics. Is this out of respect for each other's suffering? More likely it's terror. Cowed by the alarming possibilities, we regress to the status of schoolchildren in the office of the Principal. ("Maybe if we whisper, nothing bad will happen.")

After a half hour, I was moved to Doctor N's inner office, a tiny and stuffy room with a small cluttered desk and two wooden chairs. Here there were no magazines, so I did what patients do: cleared my throat, gawked about, twiddled my fingers. Nurses and receptionists padded up and down the halls, visible past the door, left ajar behind me. Tiny bottles of stuff on the shelves—samples of new drugs?—a few medical instruments (hammer for checking reflexes), bandages of various sizes, tongue depressors. It seemed bizarre to sit looking at such objects while waiting to hear how long you have to live and overhearing two nurses in the corridor discuss a third:

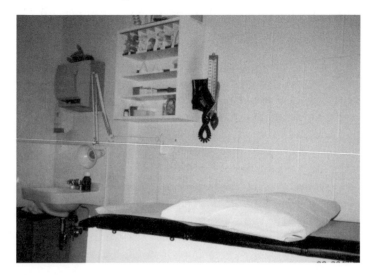

"I think we should get Louise the candles, but not the scented ones; her husband has an allergy." Christmas presents. I was wondering still if I'd make it to Christmas, my son, A's, third. To me the situation was urgent, but no one else seemed much concerned.

Eventually Doctor N joined me in the tiny office. He was a tall, somewhat fleshy man wearing a brown and green tweed jacket. He carried a file in one hand. He seemed slightly distracted but told me to stand up. I'd been sitting with my winter jacket on my lap, and in the stuffy room had begun to perspire. Also I was terrified, though a few minutes before I'd been contemplating helping myself to one of the larger bandages on the shelf nearest me: it looked perfect for those scrapes you get on your knees when you take a tumble riding a bicycle.

Doctor N poked and prodded my gut-liver area, asking questions like these: "Any pain here?" "Do you have blood in your bowel movements?" "Have you lost weight recently?" "Do you experience diarrhea?" No, no, no, no. "Facial flushing?" I was red-faced at that moment—from the warmth in the stuffy room and the stress of the interview. "Sometimes," I said, "when I drink alcohol. After sports. I play on a competitive hockey team." "Shortness of breath?" No. Here Doctor N produced a stethoscope and listened to my chest and then my liver area, and grunted.

We sat down and he looked at me for the first time since he'd introduced himself. "Well," he said flatly, "you've got cancer." I noticed he had something attached to his belt, a little black box with a wire that ran into his midriff area. I'd seen an acquaintance with fairly serious diabetes wearing something similar. Doctor N's eyes looked washed out, a washed-out brown; he looked tired. Maybe he wasn't so much distracted as in pain himself. He rolled his eyes back into focus and said, "There's not much we can do for you. There's embolization, but that's probably better saved for a little later. You seem to be doing okay now, yes?" I told him I felt fine: "I play team sports, I lead an active life."

Again Doctor N rolled his eyes as if fighting off sleep and then closed them. I thought maybe he was thinking about other carcinoid patients he'd seen, reviewing mentally his knowledge of the disease before proceeding. Then I realized that he was more than tired; he was exhausted: he might drop off at any moment. I ventured to ask, "Can you do surgery?" Doctor N roused himself. "You're stable now," he said, "and that might only stir things up." He made a motion with his hands like juggling a melon between them and added, "That might only get the malignant cells riled up and inflame them into action." No, it was better not to do that.

Now I really was sweating. I had half expected a brisk interview with an energetic and youthful practitioner who would lay out the options in front of me and suggest in a James Stewart kind of voice the most aggressive and most dangerous, but at the same time most promising, course of action: "You'll be taking a big risk, but if we go in there, we can probably clean up these tumours and have you on your feet in six months." That sort of thing. A call to arms. I'd got this idea, I realize now, from watching uplifting true life stories on American television: those programs suggest that all you need to recover from the most dreadful condition is the right (brilliant, of course) team of physicians and surgeons and the determination to get to the other side of the mountain.

What delusions we're fed—and live by!

Sleepy Doctor N said, "You've got two to five years." This was stunning news—but at least definite. I remember thinking, *good Lord, five years, A will be eight, I'll hardly have reached fifty.* Doctor N sensed my unease and continued, "Look at it this way. Everyone's going to die some time. People are killed in auto accidents and the like every day. Suddenly gone. You have this advantage over them: you know when you're going to die. You can live out your life in a kind of freedom from anxiety." In a certain way this attitude could be commended. But I confess I was not in the mood for such fatalism. Incredulous, I asked, "There's nothing can be done?"

"There is the embolization," Doctor N said, "and

somatostatin analogues when the symptoms, flushing, shortness of breath, diarrhea, become severe."

I shifted from one foot to the other. As I say, I'd expected that Doctor N would rouse me to engage in the greatest struggle of my life. I'd anticipated a girding up of the loins, excruciating sacrifices, all those resolute jaws you see on the "true story" movies and the interviews with celebrities who have survived deadly diseases. Doctor N seemed to be giving in and giving up. As I stood to leave, he extended a large moist hand and said, "Enjoy your Christmas. Enjoy your son." I think I knew before I had passed from the inner to the outer waiting room that I would never be consulting with Doctor N again.

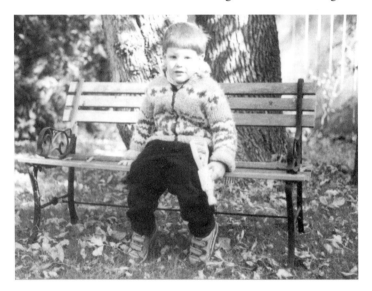

When I got home, I phoned M, our family physician. It was late in the day. "He told me I have two to five years," I informed M, adding that the prognosis had scared the crap out of me. "My goodness," M said, "that cannot be right." He sounded as astounded as I was crestfallen. "Wait one moment," M added. The line went silent. I was standing looking at the ash tree again: bare of leaves, the branches trembled in the slight movement of the chill air. This coming spring, I promised myself, we'll get that tree cut down. When M came back on the line, I heard the sound of pages being flipped. "I thought so," he said, "carcinoid syndrome. Listen. But don't take this as carved in stone." He read me a brief description of the origins and symptoms of the ailment, sentences such as these: *In 93 per cent of cases primary location of tumours is found to be in the ileum. Metastases occur in the liver, the appendix, and (rarely) the skeleton. Therapy must be directed against both tumour growth and hormone production.*

"What this all means," M explained, "is that the situation is not urgent—that is, not critical in the immediate sense. You've got time." I told him more about Doctor N and added, "I'm not happy with this prognosis, not happy at all." When I think back now on this pronouncement I feel two things: that's an arrogant thing for an inexperienced patient to assert (presumptuous anyway); and at the same time, I'm really glad I spoke out that way. It showed I was not, like Doctor N himself, prepared to give in to the conventional wisdom—to give over the struggle, you might say, and acquiesce to Death.

"You shouldn't be happy with that prognosis," M said. "Listen to this: *Unlike most metastatic neoplasms, carcinoid tumours show slow rate of growth, with patients surviving five to ten years from diagnosis.*" Five to ten years, it seemed to me, was much better than two to five. "Five years," M added, "is a long time in cancer treatment; you never know. New drugs can come along; new treatments. If you think of ten years, well, there could be a cure in ten years." I confess these were the sentiments I'd been longing to hear. I recognized they might be giving me false hope, but I was prepared to accept a degree of false hope if a prognosis also meant that my oncological team and I were prepared to actively engage carcinoid cancer.

Bernie Siegel is an oncological surgeon who writes books about how patients can best deal with cancer. Somewhere in one of his books, *Peace, Love, and Healing*, perhaps, he says that the most important thing a patient can do is be a "bad" patient. He means it this way: doctors, nurses, receptionists, the whole medical community prefer to do things in their own way, and at their pace, calling the shots on the scheduling of events, the selection of treatments to be undertaken, the amount of information provided to the patient, which other specialists are to be consulted, what hospital to book you into for a treatment, everything. A "good" patient passively accepts the paternalism implied in this arrangement, never asking questions, never daring to say, "That's inconvenient for me," and always agreeing with the doctors' perceptions and plans (though maybe unhappily), and, most important, never suggesting dissatisfaction with the attending physician, or the schedule of treatments the physician proposes. On the other hand, a "bad" patient ruffles the feathers of doctors and nurses, asking questions and consulting alternatives, for example; but in Doctor Siegel's estimation this contrary attitude forces the professionals to be more alert, more responsive, and more inventive in the care they give. In his view, as in the rap community, *bad* actually means *good.*

Moreover, asking questions, suggesting alternatives, and negotiating things such as appointments, and perhaps even treatments, involve a patient in the therapeutic process and give a patient a stake in his healing, and this may be the single most important element in survival and recovery. That is clearly the position of Walter Cannon in his famous book, *The Wisdom of the Body*: he contends that the body reacts to intrusions such as infection and disease and rights itself, that most diseases are self-terminating because the body responds to afflictions with creative adaptations. One corollary of Cannon's position is that what might be called *psychotherapeutics*, a patient's emotional disposition, is as important a factor in healing as medicines and treatments.

M and I talked for a few more minutes. He told me his father had been diagnosed with prostate cancer fifteen years earlier. "I'm prepared to believe, Wayne," he told me, "that like him, you'll die *with* your cancer but not *of* it." He said also, "I'm going to call another oncologist, so stay by the phone." I felt instantly relieved. I also knew from M's tone that I was going to be happier at the end of the day than I had been when I left Doctor N's office.

Do not misunderstand what I'm saying here. No patient of cancer or any other serious disease wants a stupidly optimistic prognosis. That would be irresponsible of a physician. But a clear-headed prognosis that also leaves something to hope for, it seems obvious, is medically responsible and humanly necessary when dealing with life-threatening diseases. We need treatment, but we also need something to believe in. It's also important to remember, as Stephen Jay Gould points out in his article about cancer ("The Median Isn't the Message"), that doctors give us average statistics when they speak of survival: since an average survival of ten years means that a certain number of patients live two years, it also means a certain number survive for eighteen years. Some patients are at the bottom end of the average, but some are at the top; you need to see yourself in the latter category. As many people know, a positive attitude makes a huge difference in surviving cancer and prolonging one's lifespan. I have seen that occur. More important, patients need to be given hope, so at the very least they can live out whatever time they have with joy in life, and not in a state of prevailing gloom.

I do not wish to belabour the point. But as patients it is well for us to remember that doctors and nurses have things going on in their lives, too, sources of distraction: family crises, financial worries, illnesses, and ailments. Some of them just do not have upbeat personalities. They might not always be in the midst of a good day when they deliver a prognosis or advice on a treatment. Their own lives, their own crises and anxieties stain what they tell us. Though they have been trained not to let such matters affect their judgement, that is a very difficult standard for them to maintain and for us to expect. So it is useful to think about your physician as you might habitually think about opinions offered to you by your family and friends, *where is this advice coming from?* No single doctor or nurse whom I've met actually meant to do anything but the best for me; but, willy-nilly, some did not do the best.

The readiness on my part to seek a second opinion or to challenge my physician has made things better for me in the long run, though it often has taken a degree of determination and a persistence that is difficult to summon up and carry out in the face of the sometimes faceless and labyrinthine medical establishment. Following diagnosis, you have to be prepared to battle, and in more ways than one.

About twenty minutes later, M called me back. He said, "I just talked to an oncologist at the Saint Boniface Hospital. I told him that you do not look ill and that you do not feel sick, and that you are in better condition than either him or me—me anyway." We both laughed. A marvellous human being and family man as well as an excellent physician, M could back off on the rich foods and take up a moderate exercise program, as he himself often says. My competitive sporting activities, I know, impressed and concerned him. "He wants to see you before the end of the week," M said, "tomorrow maybe. He feels you're going to develop a lengthy relationship. His name is Doctor KK." In my more buoyant mood I could not help thinking what a swell guy M was and how lucky I was to have such a dedicated physician in my corner— I could only hope Doctor KK would prove as committed to my improvement.

-So you want me to blame myself for contracting cancer—
"I brought it on myself"—is that the message?

-Think what you wish.

-But you do not deny it?

-Dear boy, we're looking for you to understand, to see the
conditions were ripe.

-Ripe is a positive term. Ripe means something good.

-It also means this: has come to term, is ready to undergo
something. You had run your immune system to the ground.
You'd pushed yourself to the point where you were like apples
falling from a tree.

-And this is the big thing I'm supposed to learn?—some
gobbledygook about the circumstances being favourable for the
onset of a deadly disease?

-What an attitude.

-You don't seem to grasp the fact that I'm angry—furious.

-You don't grasp the fact that we don't give a shit.

-You see, it comes to nothing, does talk. Zilch, zero, nada.

-It's your attitude that gets in the way. So unbecoming.

-Get stuffed.

-Let me start again: we aberrant cells were always here,
waiting for your body to slip into distress, into trauma.

-For the immune system to weaken.

-That's when we move in.

-Crap.

-As you will.

# Leukemia,
# Sarcoma, Liver Cancer

*There is love before, during, and after any illness.*
—John Dugdale, blind photographer with AIDS

On that awful Friday afternoon in December of 1994, K came
home from her classes at the Law School about supper time.
I told her the news. She had many questions, but I had very
few answers. We had a drink. We picked desultorily at the
food I had prepared. (It was a family maxim that whatever the
crisis, you always filled your stomach: "Keep up your
strength!") We were both stunned, moving about the house
like automatons. K offered the usual sentiments: maybe it's
not as bad as it sounds, maybe you can go to the Mayo Clinic,
let's wait and see what this oncologist (Doctor N, whom I was
to see the following week) has to say. Sane advice amidst the
sighing and fretting.

My mind was a blank, but I was restless, filled with nervous energy that had no outlet. K suggested we go for a walk.
Despite the cold of December and the wind blowing from the
north, that was a good suggestion: the stars had never seemed
so bright, the air so invigorating. I recalled that when A was a
tiny baby (born in February), I had taken him out for walks

on frosty evenings such as this one, bundled up in a Snugli and buttoned under a heavy leather team jacket I wore in those days, our two hearts beating in close proximity, as his foetal heart had at one time beat with his mother's. K told me we had to be strong, we had to have a positive attitude, and that we'd get through whatever was coming. More typical stuff. She also said she was going to get in touch with an herbalist the next day, and begin to pursue alternative forms of therapy. My mother had been ingesting a powerful health drink, K recalled (The Missing Link); maybe it and other similar products could be employed against the cancer. I was grateful for K's matter-of-fact tone, her readiness to think about things in a positive way, her specific suggestions; but I was also deep in that state of blankness where you're only half-hearing things that are being said to you and not absorbing much of what you do take in.

"I'm shattered," I said. "What will happen to A?"

"He'll be all right," K said, "children are amazingly resilient. It's you we have to worry about."

I tried not to have those self-pitying thoughts about the unfairness of life, or to spit out the words, *you're talking to a dead man.*

Halfway through our walk, which we were making mostly in stunned silence, K said, "Call your sisters."

I asked my younger sister, C, if she was alone and could spare a few minutes (she's the mother of four, two of whom were toddlers at the time). Almost before I said, "I've got cancer," we both started to weep. That was okay. I'd been suppressing a cauldron of emotions and felt like one of those overfilled tankers you see on animated cartoons, rivets popping and about to explode. The release through tears was healthy. We both knew the family history well enough not to need to recur to it: two aunts succumbed to leukemia in their fifties; another uncle died of a cancer in his liver at age sixty-two. Our paternal grandmother had suffered a lengthy battle with an intestinal cancer in the 1950s. (Our parents had both come from families of seven children, so that made twelve sets of aunts and uncles; we were part of a group of twenty-eight first cousins, two of whom had died at their own hands quite young.) When our tears had passed we talked quietly for some time, agreeing that this was not the time to tell our mother, who at that point had suffered from a weak heart for more than a decade. C said, "If there's anything I can say, anything at all that I can do." But there wasn't.

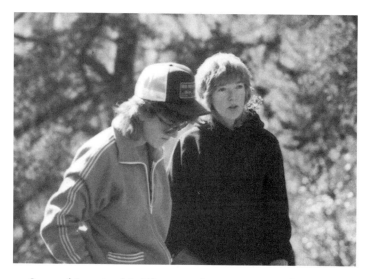

Some things in this life come down to you and you alone. As a child, you have to learn how to balance a two-wheeler on your own, because no one can do that for you; as a teen, you have to dial the numbers and say into the receiver in your own voice, "May I speak to Susie, please." When you become an adult, especially one with a terminal ailment, you have to stand on the brink of the wide abyss, as the poet says, and think about your fate until "Love and Fame to nothingness do shrink." You are alone. Others can be there with us; others can hold our hands; others may mutter the words we humans say to each other to help us through these moments of crisis and despair. But soon comes the silence; soon comes the lying in the dark alone looking at the pattern in the ceiling tiles; some roads, ultimately, you have to walk down alone.

My elder sister wanted details. She was angry that Doctor MF had given me no idea what treatments were in store for me, no prognosis, nothing but that flat statement, *you have cancer.* Ordinarily the more quiet of my two sisters, she's faced a lot of difficulties in her own life—raising two children by herself—and has triumphed in ways that are remarkable. She's also one of those "When she was good, she was very, very good" types; look out, though, if you cross her. Like my sister C, she wept a bit, too, but she was thinking almost immediately about what we could do. "I'm going to call my friend— a physician—in Victoria," she said, "and find out about this carcinoid thing." She had me spell it out as best I could guess. She refused to believe that there were not many avenues of redress available, and she insisted I take that approach, too. "I'm going to make some inquiries on Monday," she declared firmly. "There's new drugs, they do surgeries on all cancers now; there's got to be something that can be done." She'd heard of specialized cancer clinics in the USA and of alternative health practices. Her go-get-'em attitude and the determination in her voice were heartening. We acquire hope from all kinds of things: from a touch at the right moment, from commiseration, from people reminding us that most survivors of cancer have had the determination to beat it and a positive attitude. The readiness of loved ones to take up the issue for us, to shoulder some of the weight, ranks very high in the list.

"I know this isn't easy to do," S told me before she hung up, "but don't get worked up about this before you know what's involved. We're all here for you. We'll borrow money from the estate if we have to and get you the best treatment there is." Like K she was thinking ahead, to the time when expensive treatments might be necessary. I was still in such a funk that I had never considered that money might be an issue.

K gave me a shoulder rub. We had been visiting a massage therapist, EB, for years, a man who had helped us both through difficult emotional times, and after she was done rubbing me, she said, "Make an appointment with EB first thing Monday." Intuitively she knew that I needed his strong hands and calming presence. I slept better than I had imagined would be possible. Nervous exhaustion led to prostration.

The next afternoon, my sister S showed up at the door with a bottle of wine and a paperback book, Carl O. Simonton's *Getting Well Again*. Simonton, she reported, ran a famous cancer recovery clinic in the United States. His book outlined some of the procedures they employed at that institution and some of the advice they gave the newly diagnosed. My sister pressed these items on me. She had driven to our neighbourhood from her own in her ageing and rust-pocked sedan: I could hear its motor ticking over in the lane as she talked. She did not stay long but she said, "Read the book. If nothing else, you'll feel better. Somebody else has been down this road and

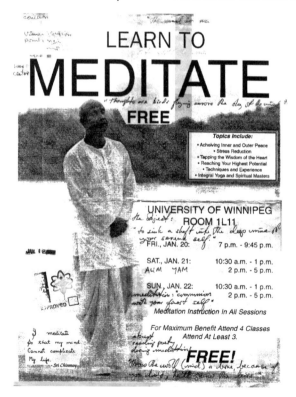

come through at the far end." She looked at me directly and soberly—and then winked! She had a folded flyer in her purse. It was printed on blue paper and read, "Learn To Meditate Free!" In addition to concluding that my sister was a wonderful person, I felt something akin to the ground shifting under my feet. A child of the fifties, I had been raised to expect certain things of myself as a man—authority and courage, among them. Within my nuclear family I had been the conventional success story. Though they each had had their share of successes, my sisters had by-and-large looked to me for leadership in the family; even my father had sought out my counsel at important moments. So it was unusual for me to be the fragile member of the group, the one needing solace, the one receiving help and advice. The weak link. I recognized dimly that I was embarking on a new role in life.

I gave my sister a hug and promised to read the book. About the meditation I also thought, *what the hell*. The classes began after Christmas.

-My friend died.

-This tone is unbecoming.

-My friend is dead and you killed her.

-Oh, more accusations, dear boy.

-Shut up and listen: dead at thirty-two.

-Perhaps she learned something about herself before dying, perhaps—

-Listen. She called me on the telephone. They had removed a tumour from her tongue and throat. She could barely talk. But she was filled with hope and looking forward to a surgery in Texas. She believed, she wanted to believe in life. It was awful.

-You're hysterical.

-She was beautiful. She was only thirty-two. Loved scuba diving. Her zest for life sparkled in her eyes. She was joyful and life-affirming. She had borne a son only a year earlier.

-Listen, sometimes a hormone imbalance occurs following childbirth, and then—

-No, you listen. She loved life; she was a good mother; she made people laugh.

-You cannot know what was really going on in her life.

-I know she loved her child and her husband and her friends and her work, and now she's fucking dead.

-These are the ravings of a spoiled child. Quite unbecoming.

-I hate these words of yours: *My boy, so unbecoming.* I loathe your superior airs. Your tone disgusts me. Even more, I despise what you stand for.

-And what is that, pray?

-Smarmy intellectual rationalizations of brute facts. You're the Doctor Goebbels of the Oncology Ward.

-Oh dear. Such bile. And I thought we were making progress.

-Piss off.

-Dear boy, you're becoming irrational.

-I have every right to be fucking irrational. CP is dead! You killed her.

-As you will.

# Shark Cartilage and Essiac

*A person seldom falls sick but the bystanders are*
*animated with a faint hope that he will die.*
                              —Ralph Waldo Emerson

1.

About a week after I told my sisters about the cancer, I was
talking with my friend, D, on the telephone. We'd been colleagues at the university years earlier. He still taught there.
Inevitably he asked, "How are you keeping?" This was a tricky
moment. Over all the years we'd known each other, almost
twenty, we'd maintained a conventional male friendship,
steady but reserved support for each other through marital and
career crises of various kinds. We'd had a few Scotches and
downed our share of draft beer in our time; typically, though,
men of our generation and background (Nordic) do not wear
their hearts on their sleeves. But something was beginning to
change in me in that regard, as well as in others. So I told him.
   "Good God," he said. "What's it called again?" He fumbled
on the other end of the line for a pen and then had me spell
out carcinoid syndrome. "My nephew, KT," he said, "works

for a drug company. Maybe he knows something, maybe he can help. You remember KT?" I did. We had chatted several times over drinks in the bar; he was a nice fellow who had turned from a bright career in medical surgery to working for a large pharmaceutical interest. But what can an ordinary guy, however nice, who works for a drug company do for a victim of cancer?

KT, it turned out, was anything but an ordinary guy.

The next evening, another blustery and cold prairie night, D appeared at the door of our house, his long white hair and beard dishevelled in the swirling wind. A man approaching sixty, he stands well over six feet and perfectly defines the term *mesomorph*: a man who fills a doorway with his presence and a room with his personality. He had two large binders clutched to his chest. "I'm not coming in," he said, "but KT wanted you to have these. Don't be afraid of them. Read them. He says you have contracted an unusual cancer, but it's not a rampant variety and can be controlled with a drug that may afford you many years." He offered me the binders, slippery plastic things, bulky and weighty, jammed full of medical reports on carcinoid cancer, perhaps five hundred pages of reading material in total.

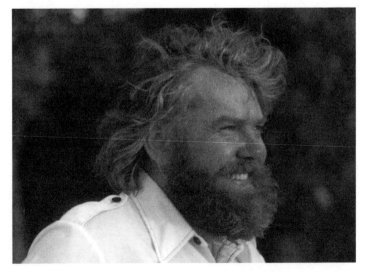

I took them into the house and plunked them on my desk. Reading all that stuff would have seemed a formidable task at the best of times. When you've been diagnosed with a life-threatening disease, that taxing discovery and the anxiety that follows can sap you of energy. Just getting through an ordinary day in the first few weeks may be about all you can manage: you tend toward listlessness. So you can find masses of reading a daunting prospect. I think this is why Carl Simonton in one of his books suggests that cancer patients have a "team," a small support group of healthy family and friends, who read things before patients do, minimizing, so to speak, the workload of familiarizing oneself with one's ailment. (Simonton also suggests that whenever possible a member of a patient's team—a spouse or adult child—speak on the telephone with doctors and others in the medical domain, again lowering the stress factor for the patient: functioning as a buffer zone.) This is sound advice. Dealing with the physical aspects of one's condition is a draining task; add to that the psychological labyrinth one is negotiating—fears and anxieties about pain, about one's lifespan, about the loss of career, the impact on family—and a patient has to be an unusual specimen not to be constantly strung out and worn down. This is particularly true in the first six months or so after diagnosis.

When my sister S had brought me over Simonton's books, I had put them on my bedside reading table. When my friend MD had given me Norman Cousins's *Anatomy of an Illness,* I had thanked him and marked it for immediate attention, too. When a nephew brought me over articles on shark cartilage and Essiac, I read them and discussed with K the possibility of acquiring some of each. Everyone was being very helpful. But I could see that having cancer was becoming a new career for me, a study, a life-undertaking. There was going to be little time for hand-wringing and self-pity.

A few mornings later I began flipping through the binders D had brought me. There were glossy brochures describing various pancreatic and liver cancers, endocrine tumours—

with full-colour illustrations of lesions and tumours. This graphic stuff is not for the faint of heart. ("Gross section of the ileum with multiple small carcinoids in the mucosa: note the discoid appearance of some of the tumours.") Certain statements and phrases leapt out of these publications: "In our experience with 103 patients, 39 died during an eight-year observation period." And: "Complete remissions have only occasionally been seen." Such statements plunge you into a downward spiral. Phrases sometimes cause one to flutter with anxiety: *cervical neoplasia, squamous cell skin carcinoma, malignant melanoma.* Lovely words, in a way, musical, but frightening, too. I marked off passages in highlighter pen for later study and tried not to think of the sections entitled Mortality, Side Effects, Autoimmune Disease, Death. Information,

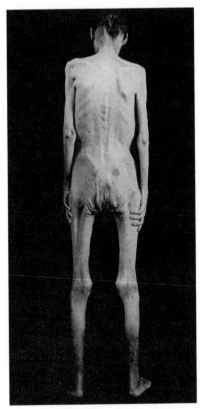

though, is never in itself a bad thing, and when I emerged from the binders a week or so later ("a sadder and a wiser man," as a poet once put it), I had a pretty good notion about how carcinoid cancer begins, how it develops from inception to mortality, incidence of morbidity, and which methods of treatment had so far produced encouraging results.

D called and spoke with me briefly. Since he'd given me the binders, he had been concerned that I might have been overwhelmed, perhaps to the point of depression, and was relieved to hear that overall I felt better for having read the detailed and exotic language of the medical journals KT had gathered up for me. I felt the knowledge I had gained had put me in a stronger position regarding the cancer in me. Maybe knowing the general parameters of the disease would better equip me to face the worst aspects of the physical changes that were coming and at the same time enable me to discuss intelligently with my physicians the treatments and alternatives that were possible. However shaken by my prospects for an ordinary lifespan, I was inclined to agree with something Francis Bacon once said: "Knowledge is Power."

"Thanks, D," I said. "Light is better than darkness." By this juncture the Christmas season had passed. Soon afterwards, K and A and I travelled to Mexico and splashed in the ocean and lay in the sun for two weeks, drinking Sol beer and Cuba Libras, and the weight that had lain heavily on all of us since mid-December lifted. When we returned home, K spent some time reading books about eating habits and neuropathy, and she spoke at length with an uncle in Vancouver who had changed his dietary regimen after being diagnosed with a cancer that had subsequently ebbed into remission. We were planning on visiting an herbalist; I was going to take the course in meditation in early February and was looking forward to that experience.

One day not long after our return home there was a message on the answering machine from KT, asking me to call him. Before I had properly thanked him for the binders he'd sent along with D, he announced that he'd arranged for Doctor KO to come to visit the oncological community in Winnipeg and to review my case with my physicians and me. At first I could not take this information in: Doctor KO is the world's foremost authority on carcinoid cancer. His clinic in Uppsala, Sweden, does the most advanced research and treatment on neoendocrine and carcinoid tumours. He has the widest experience of any physician with carcinoid patients— and over the longest period of time. KT said, "Doctor KO will be here March the fifth and he would like to meet you."

In the following weeks I spent a lot of hours reviewing

Doctor KO's articles: I wanted to be familiar with his case studies and to have facts at my command. A visit to the library at the medical college and a few hours with the Internet engine Med-Line armed me with a wealth of information about the disease and treatment trials.

At the appointed time I found myself sitting in a lecture theatre at the medical college with perhaps twenty oncologists. Some were taking notes; others just listening, as I was. Everyone but KT and I and Doctor KO wore a white smock. Doctor KO, who spoke that immaculate English one learns from British schoolmasters abroad, gave a straightforward, professional, and precise outline of the etiology and symptomology of carcinoid syndrome. He'd come equipped with a slide presentation—more somewhat gruesome illustrations of diseased organs—that included numerous graphs and charts. His presentation lasted almost an hour. Questions followed. I did not have the courage to pose the few I had. Then KT, who'd introduced Doctor KO, sidled over to where I was sitting and pointed out that a video was being made of the presentation and that I was welcome to have a copy if I wished. I did. KT said he would arrange it.

Later in the day at another location, Doctor KO reviewed my case history in my presence and that of a select group of oncologists, including Doctor KK. It felt odd to see my insides on a giant projector screen, and to have doctors KK and KO pointing to places on a cross-section of my liver and discussing the progress of the disease and the possible remedies for it. At the conclusion of a brief presentation, Doctor KO noted that I was present in the room; a ripple of appreciation mixed with mild bemusement ran through the smock-suited physicians. "Do you have any questions?" Doctor KO wanted to know from me. I asked if it was okay to drink wine. "If that's what you were doing before, of course," he said, "enjoy yourself, enjoy your life." I grew more bold and asked, "What is the longest time any patient of yours has survived with carcinoid syndrome?" Doctor KO twinkled and said in his immaculate English, "A man we diagnosed in 1984 is doing well and looking forward to many more years."

After the meeting broke up, we shook hands. Doctors KK and KO had more to discuss. KT gave me the tape he'd had made of the earlier presentation. He said he had made notes from the discussion of my case history and would mail me a summary. I left the medical college buoyed up in many ways. Meeting Doctor KO was only the most obvious of these. Hearing him discuss my case and use phrases such as "superior general health," "encouraging early diagnosis," and "excellent prospects" were just the thing I needed in the early phases of my diagnosis. There had been many days when I'd bemoaned my dismal prospects for reaching sixty, for seeing my son graduate from high school, so this one was a welcome counter-balance.

At home that night I told K about the day's events. "There's a light in your face," she said, "that I haven't seen there for many months." It was not only my face that was light. For a number of weeks I felt physically lifted. Perhaps I'm one of those born sanguine optimists and would have taken up the issue with this disease whatever else occurred. But the visit of Doctor KO filled me with optimism and charged me with an enormous energy that continues to this day. The world authority on my disease was on my side, on my extended team.

I cannot say enough in praise of KT. He'd given me all that reading material and assumed I could handle the contents and ramifications. He had not talked down to me about the disease or about the drug Doctor KO recommended I take to combat it: a biological modifier called Alpha Interferon 2b. He had gone out of his way to arrange the visit of Doctor KO. I was, after all, merely an acquaintance from the bar. He'd made sure I was in the audience on the day of Doctor KO's talk, and had given me, as well as the video recording of the presentation, a concise summary of Doctor KO's observations about my case—and his recommendations for treatment. After the event, he spoke to me on the phone and fielded a dozen questions I was too embarrassed to ask in the presence of the oncologists. A week or so later I met D for coffee. I told him I thought KT was a saint. "Without exaggeration," I said, "he's given me the hope to go on." I was not saying this just to make D feel good about his nephew: family, friends, acquaintances who are willing to go to bat for us in our distress are absolutely critical to our survival and recovery. We not only can benefit from a team, we need one; and the more we can do to acquire one, the better off we can be. So I repeated to D, despite my usual aversion to terms such as *genius* and *masterpiece,* and so on, "KT is a saint."

As I say, we're not given to demonstrations of emotion or speaking sentimentally. D said softly, "He's a wonderful man, KT." He had to steady his mug of coffee with both hands before drinking; then we moved on to other subjects.

## 2.

Friends help us by finding things out for us in the newspapers or magazines or on the television; they also sometimes bring things to us that may help in the treatments we are undertaking: news items, publications, alternate remedies. They act on our behalf, researching the Internet, say, or consulting a physician in another area of specialty. These are direct interventions in our therapy, and very useful ones; D and KT are exemplary in this regard. But friends serve a much broader, though indirect, function when we're suffering from a life-threatening disease.

Some years ago a medical journalist named Norman Cousins was diagnosed with a rare disease: his cells were almost literally falling apart from a collagen illness. Perhaps today we would call this the "flesh eating disease." Whatever the case, Cousins took two immediate steps to deal with his condition. Following the lead of Linus Pauling, Cousins began immediately to ingest massive doses of Vitamin C, an antioxidant that inhibits the function of the free radicals that break down cell homogeneity. This was a direct physiological intervention. The second thing Cousins did was rather less organic: from the time he was a teenager a lover of the Marx

Brothers, he brought into his hospital room all of their movies and watched at least one every day. He was, as he put it in his book, *Anatomy of an Illness,* trying to laugh himself back to health. And he succeeded.

Laughter is a powerful curative. In order to laugh we have to be distracted—or is it more accurate to say that we have to become so focussed on a humorous situation that we momentarily forget all others? Patients of terminal diseases tend to become wrapped up in them—consciously and unconsciously worrying about what is happening inside their bodies. Laughter breaks through this cocoon of anxiety that we spin around ourselves. For a short period we come out of ourselves. Laughter also reminds us that this life is a great comedy, that there is always something to smile at or chuckle about, that enjoying each moment as it unfolds is one way to live a life. In brief, it frees us from the mental baggage we carry around concerning our "case." It is also physical release. To laugh, you have to let go with your muscles. And whether you realize it or not, as a victim of a life-threatening disease, you expend a lot of muscle energy (conscious and unconscious) on tightening up. We rigidify with anxiety and dread. In addition, we make ourselves into clenched fists of determination; we're intent on

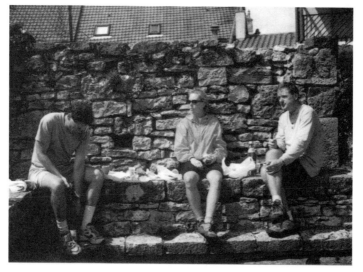

defeating the bad thing inside us. We bunch up our muscles, especially those in the torso and neck and stomach, to meet the challenge of the disease, making our bodies into hard little resistant balls against the affliction, armadillo-like. But sometimes we need to let go, and laughter provides us with a perfect avenue for such releases. Norman Cousins actually did laugh himself back to health. His manic strategy is perhaps not for everyone, but it's certainly worth a shot.

Friends serve a similar indirect function. Friends meet us and talk to us about subjects of global interest that are not our health. Friends remind us of past experiences when we shared a laugh or undertook a foolhardy task that looks from another point in time as madcap as the contrived foolishness on television sitcoms. One of my friends, R, meets me regularly for breakfast and we share an hour of chat, laughing, teasing each other, and re-living our past histories. We've known each other since high school. He has had a brother and a brother-in-law die of cancer: so he's gone through two dissimilar but equally revelatory experiences with cancer and subsequent death. When he speaks about them, he fingers his chin, choosing his words carefully. He's sensitive, non-judgemental, and wise. He gives me perspective. He offers me priceless advice.

Friends tell us jokes. Friends engage us in intense conversations about the things that matter to us—in my case, the arts, literature, writers, and sports. They take us out of ourselves into the things that energize and enrich our lives. Friends do things with us: a friend and I plan to travel to Florida next spring to witness baseball's annual rite of spring training. In short, friends are the agents by which we engage life—in the case of cancer patients, re-engage life.

Major changes may occur when you have a life-threatening disease. Significant changes *do* occur. No one who has been diagnosed with cancer is ever the same afterwards. We become more thoughtful; we become more aware of our mortality; we cherish loved ones and become more forgiving of their foibles—and of our own. Most days now I look in the mirror as I brush my teeth and see a man I would not have recognized

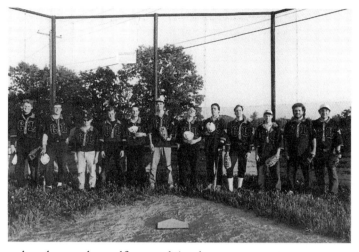

a decade ago: less self-assured (perhaps *arrogant* is more accurate) than in my twenties, but also more knowledgeable about life and content within myself. We also become short-tempered; we sense the building up of anger inside ourselves; we may become dark and moody; we may become more skeptical than we were before—or even cynical at times, perceiving life in a darker shade. Our friends sense these things. All of them become aware that we are not the same as we once were; some of them try to help us over the bumpy spots; most see that the dynamic of the relationship shared between us before diagnosis has changed and will continue to change as we wrestle with our pain and our mortality; a few become confused, and, not knowing how to cope with the changes in us, turn away from us. That is very sad; friends should stick by us, we feel; but it's probably more important to keep focussed on the major issue, one's health, than it is to fester about the loss of a single friend who is not up to the challenge of re-inventing the friendship.

If friends are critically important to cancer patients, they are equally valuable to relatives and spouses of cancer sufferers. Everyone associated with a cancer victim has bad days—anxieties, fears, depressions, loss of faith. Cancer victims are granted the right to rant, to weep, to curse their gods and their bad fortune: to slam doors, to scream in outrage and howl at life's inequity. I've behaved atrociously on a number of occasions since diagnosis. Perhaps everyone does. Once when I was at a clinic I witnessed a memorable incident. In the consulting room next to the one I occupied, waiting for my oncologist, an older woman patient went ballistic: she screamed at her physician, threw objects about the room, screeched "bastard," and finally wailed in despair. Her daughter, who was accompanying her, tried to comfort the woman, and for her pains was called "meddling slut." I recall sitting very still through the woman's rant; sweat broke out on the backs of my hands and ran down my forehead. I remembered my own fury on occasions, and I also recall thinking this is not a bad thing, sometimes there is nothing to do, really, except wail like a wounded animal. Yet whereas cancer patients are allowed to vent their angers, the spouses of patients are required to be the constant shoulder to cry on, the voice of reason, and the champion of hope. It's unrealistic to expect this exemplary behaviour from anyone, so friends are an invaluable resource to spouses and other people going through the struggle with us: to those friends of their own, our spouses and relatives can voice their alarm, reveal their despondency, weep at their own helplessness, and so on (even, from time to time, curse the cancer patient, who has encumbered them with a terrible burden of their own). These are all legitimate human frailties they cannot reveal in front of the cancer victim. It might be particularly useful for a spouse to have a friend—or develop one—who is going through a similar experience. We all need support in this business, and solid, sane, calm friends can be a source of strength for both patients and those closest to them.

-So, my boy, it's been a while. You've been sulking?

-I've been meditating, trying to understand what you meant by another way of seeing—another way of seeing the reason that you came along.

-Let me say again: we came to develop, to flourish.

-Ugh. I hate your sophistry, your verbal pyrotechnics. *Ripe, flourish.*

-OK. There are things we hate about you. But at least you're calm today. So let's get on with it.

-OK. The fact that you've infested me—

-No name-calling, correct? No tantrums.

-OK. The fact that you are here changes things, yes. I have had to re-assess my life.

-Yes. You had to recognize that you are not immortal. And you had to stop living the way you were living.

-I admit that much. I have had to limit drinking, say, and to change eating habits and stop abusing my body with weird hours and dubious foods: Cokes, barbecued wings, processed foods, alcohol.

-See. Live better, in other words.

-Christ almighty! You want to take the credit for that?

-For anything and everything that you concede.

-What I see is crap and bullshit.

-Such adolescent ranting, really. But you admit you've learned something, you've grown.

-I don't want to admit it. But in some small ways I now know myself better.

-"In some small ways"?

-I have had to slow the pace of my life; I have had to re-examine myself. There were things I believed and things I did that I had to re-assess, step back from and admit were not the only way to do things—to see things. I've had to think about mortality, my own and that of others. I have had to think of the world—of my loved ones—going on into time without me. That is a painful thought. We want to live. For humans to live is all. I have had to ponder what I have done and what I am.

-Next you'll be saying you understand the meaning of life.

-You piss me off, you know? You say I have an attitude but then I get this crap from you.

-I only made a cliché of your observation.

-And I only acknowledged that I have had to look inside myself.

-OK. You've looked inside yourself; you've grown.

# Octreotide and Pigs' Hearts

*Each patient carries his own doctor inside him.*
—Albert Schweitzer

One of the truly amazing things about contemporary life is that you can instantly be in touch with people worldwide who are suffering from the same disease as you are. Almost immediately after I was diagnosed, my friend D called me on the telephone and asked, "You have access to the Web, don't you?" I did, but then, in 1994, I had little idea how to go about using it to my full advantage. Which I confessed to D. "Come down to my office," he said, "and we'll see what we can do."

I did. We punched in *carcinoid syndrome*, or *gastrointestinal cancer*, or some such coordinates, and in a few minutes—it was a wonder to me then and remains so now—up popped the name of T, an Australian woman who had herself just been diagnosed with carcinoid cancer and was looking to connect with fellow sufferers. We sent messages forth and back. She told me that she taught at a college where she lived, that she had a teenage daughter, and that she wanted to share information with carcinoid patients. We swapped details about our cases: when we were diagnosed, where we were on the "curve" of the disease, what treatments we had taken already and anticipated taking in the future.

This was all exciting—and more important, reassuring—for me. T was the first actual person I knew of who had contracted the relatively rare cancer I had. We were fellow sufferers, two who could say, "I have this disease in my gut and liver and I feel such-and-such about it." No one close to you can share in quite that way. So relief and satisfaction. Somewhere into our second or third set of e-mails, T asked, "Do you know of JM?" I didn't. JM's mother had been a carcinoid patient, diagnosed later in life. JM saw her through her final years; but JM had not been content to stand by and passively watch her mother succumb to cancer. In addition to leading an active work life and providing solace to her ailing mother, JM had made herself into an e-conduit for carcinoid patients. An American, she was in touch with sufferers worldwide; more, she knew the e-mail addresses and telephone numbers of oncologists all over the USA; even more than that, she had coordinated a telephone chat-line for patients of carcinoid cancer: if you dialled a certain number and punched in a secret code, you could join an open-line free-for-all gabfest on the second Saturday evening of every month, starting at eight o'clock.

JM was very upbeat. E-mailing me, she wrote things like, "Howdy, Wayne, glad to have you on board." She gave me a list of e-mail addresses and access to dozens of other carcinoid patients, with whom I initially shared information on treatments and in time discussed how it felt to be a cancer patient. Shortly after I hooked up with JM's circle, for example, B wrote to say he was going into hospital for an operation on his liver. DD wrote to him, saying, "We're looking forward to hearing from you on Wednesday"—the day following B's surgery. SA wrote to B, "Keep the faith. Remember E went through this last year and came out better than she went in." I recall it was all a bit touchy-feely to my thinking—back-slapping and encouragement to someone you'd never met or even seen. I'd grown up in a world, my father's, defined by advice like *Never let down your guard, never show them weakness* ("them" being the other team, the boss, the banks, the government, and so on). But I managed to add my hesitant voice to the group: "Good luck, B." And I'm glad I did. He wrote back the following Thursday: "I'm weak, so I'll keep this short. Thanks, Wayne. When I went in for the surgery, it was like you were all standing round the gurney holding my hand. Every little bit helps."

JM put me in touch with two men she thought might have more in common with me than the dozens of other carcinoid sufferers connected to her group. V was a thirty-two-year-old schoolteacher with aspirations to be a writer. He lived on the eastern seaboard of the USA with his wife. They were debating whether to have children, a difficult decision when you have a life-threatening disease. V's situation was more serious than my own. He had been diagnosed when he began to suffer chest pains: the valves in his heart had begun to deteriorate as a result of the hormone/peptide activity of his tumours. He had recently had a valve replaced with the valve from a pig's heart, but that had not gone as well as might have been hoped; that valve, too, was fast deteriorating, and V was anticipating a second operation, again to receive a pig's valve replacement. Still, he was keeping the faith, continuing to teach, and beginning to write a book about his home town, Baltimore. By e-mail he told me he disliked having to inject himself two or three times a day with octreotide, a symptom depressor. "I hate it," he wrote, "but what the hay?"

L lived somewhere in Montana. He was in his early forties, a lawyer, who, with his wife, was raising two adopted Oriental girls. Like V's, his condition was further advanced than mine. He experienced bad flushing and severe diarrhea and needed to inject octreotide subcutaneously three or more times during the work day. He was doing this secretly. He had not told anyone at his place of work that he had cancer. He had not told his two school-age girls. I did not find this surprising (*Don't let down your guard, don't show them weakness*), though I did—and do—think of secrecy as a less positive way of dealing with cancer than others. Disclosure. Facing up to it.

When I was younger I might have thought similarly to L:

that my personal life should not cross over with my professional life. We've been taught this. You have two parallel tracks that make up your existence, but they should not become tangled up. A wag in a change room once put it this way: *Don't shit where you eat.* Possibly this is the way most men think about their lives, young men, anyway. Perhaps they think that revealing such things is also revealing weakness, or asking for pity; it isn't. So I think of disclosure differently now. It's all your personal life, isn't it? And not admitting that you're a victim of disease, a sufferer, that you're frail, is denying it, is pretending that this terrible—I use the word advisedly—chain of events is not happening to you. Is that really the way to deal with such a critical life experience?

Still. One of the things you learn quickly when you have a terminal disease is that everyone handles issues such as disclosure and involvement in treatments differently. L is entitled to his secretiveness as much as Bill is entitled to his candour.

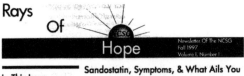

## Rays Of Hope

Newsletter Of The NCSG
Fall 1997
Volume I, Number I

### In This Issue...

### Sandostatin, Symptoms, & What Ails You

Sandostatin—most of us are on this drug to control the symptoms of the carcinoid syndrome: diarrhea, flushing, and wheezing. But what do we know about this drug? Well, we all know one thing: it's *expensive!* The good news is that there are new forms coming to market, one which should be cheaper, and researchers continue to tinker to improve the drug.

The basic drug that we use is called Sandostatin, named after the drug company that developed it, Sandoz Pharmaceuticals. (After a corporate merger, the company changed its name to Novartis.) Sandostatin is the *trade* name for the drug octreotide; octreotide is the generic name. Octreotide itself is but one form of the parent drug, somatostatin. Therefore, octreotide is but one of many forms of somatostatin. (In "Doctor Speak," it's a somatostatin *analogue*.) These artificial forms of somatostatin are not foreign to our bodies, for they try to mimic our body's *own natural* somatostatin.

### On To The Hormones

But how does Sandostatin work? First, we must understand our tumors.

Carcinoid tumors are strange buggers in many ways. Like tumors in other forms of cancer, carcinoid tumors do grow. But carcinoid tumors have another "trick"—they produce a rich brew of hormones, each which your tumor may or may not produce, and each of which may or may not produce side effects. Some of these substances are:

- serotonin
- substance P
- chromogranin A
- histamine
- enkephalin
- dopamine
- kallikrein
- prostaglandin
- neurotensin
- neurokinin A & neurokinin B
- neuropeptide K & neuropeptide Y
- motilin
- gastrin releasing peptide (GRP)
- ACTH
- VIP
- & More!

*continued on page 4* ▶

Here's an interesting thing. About two years after I first made contact with T, I lost contact with her. Despite posting repeated e-mail messages, I did not receive a response. Was she undergoing a treatment, or recovering from surgery and too weak to sit at her computer keyboard—or worse? I contacted JM. "What's happened to T?" I asked, fearful of what JM might tell me. But T had not died. JM wrote: "T is now denying that she has cancer. She's broken off communication."

Go figure. T was my first contact with the carcinoid circle that JM coordinated, that initial lifeline so essential in helping a cancer sufferer to regain emotional balance. She gave me hope and put me in touch with JM's active and supportive "Rays of Hope" group. When I heard she'd dropped out, it disturbed me that she had taken the course she had, but her behaviour, like L's, did not surprise me. Dealing with a life-threatening illness is wearing, physically and psychologically. Sometimes some people need a *time out* of sorts, a period to *not* be victims, to not be daily fighting the good fight, to not be trekking into clinics and suffering through injections and scans and radiation pictures and God knows what all else: chatting with other patients by e-mail, for example. I hope T comes back to all that some day soon, renewed and rejuvenated in a way that will allow her to enjoin the battle afresh; but I'll understand if she doesn't.

After the initial period of intense e-mail activity, which lasted several years, I myself backed off those communications for a while: too much "chatting," too many jokes, too much correspondence of a not-very-personal or helpful nature. (This was 1997 or so, when it was still common to open up your e-mail application in the morning and discover that dozens of messages had been dumped into your system overnight.)

Over the years I've kept up an informative and humorous exchange with a Swedish man named J. He has lived with carcinoid syndrome for nearly two decades. In our many e-chats J seemed generous, good-humoured, and intelligent, and always willing to share information about his case and offer encouragement about mine. For years he's acted as secretary of

CARPA, the Carcinoid Patients' Association: he regularly mails out an information bulletin about treatments and drugs. Our discussions have been lively and useful. J's English is touch-and-go, but my Swedish is non-existent. Still, we get our messages across. From his side, he's experienced most of the treatments that European physicians employ with carcinoid patients: he knows a lot about interferons, for instance. From my side, I've had the unusual radio-isotope treatment, discussed in a later chapter. As a result of our e-mail friendship, we know more about our mutual disease, and we share stuff about being cancer patients that is more personal: family things, fears, hopes. I've been glad of his friendship.

In the meantime, I've re-established contact with SA, with whom I had been in contact in the mid-nineties. She had a great deal of information to pass along to me by way of the Internet. In that regard, things had changed in the year or so since I'd been intensely involved in e-friendships. SA had her own home page where she'd briefly outlined her cancer journey: "My Story," it's called. A number of other patients with carcinoid cancer had similar home pages. I spent a busy weekend or two getting back in touch with other patients—and with JM, who had begun running the National Carcinoid Support Group. People were active; patients felt positive about their prospects and those of all carcinoid patients; good things were happening.

Here's another curious thing: the e-mail relationship has not been wholly positive. The heartening experience of cheering on B and then hearing back from him after his successful surgery was balanced by having E's husband, P, e-mail us from their home in England to say she died following a period of suffering and struggle. The daily jokes PJ posted us were balanced by IT writing me, "I'm a biologist so I know what's coming for us; this little critter is nasty and I'm not looking forward to what the ugly bugger's going to do to us some day soon."

Finally, the e-mail friendships end. After five years of correspondence, I began to hear less and less from V and L. At the time of writing, I have not heard from either of them for over a year. T has disappeared from the Internet, claiming she is not

---

**In memoriam**

*Jarl Jacobson*

After 20 years as a carcinoid patient, Jarl Jacobson has left us. Jarl was one of the co-founders of CARPA. He lived long enough to to take part in CARPA´s 10 years anniversary CARPAs 10 years anniversary, which was, due to the circumstances, celebrated within a small number of people in Norrbotten, Sweden. During the period since CARPA started, Jarl has been its driving force and enthusiast, whom without his great commitment, the association would not exist.

Jarl edited the CARPA-bulletin and was treasurer of the association. He took care of all the member files and held contact with members, in Sweden as well as internationally; all this work he managed to carry out from his small office under a staircase in his home.

Jarl showed a certain talent in recruiting new members, a talent, which was a part of a mind opening and frank nature. Jarl especially cared for the founding of a contact network within the association He himself acted in this direction, he listened and was always available for the members and their problems. His commitment in CARPA Jarl carried out with enthusiasm and idealism. Besides CARPA Jarl also put a lot of engagement in other activities and was for example during several years the driving force in Norrbotten´s local "Hem och Skolaförening", an association for parents elucidating school children´s interests.

At an early stage of my sickness, I had the privilege of getting to know Jarl, and he became a friend, a brother patient with time for the troubles and sorrows of others. I also got to know his family and it stood clear to me what a loving and caring father Jarl was. In spite of his disease, Jarl supported his sons in their practice of sports.

A lasting memory of Jarl is the memory of a man with a great and human commitment he never had to talk about. Instead Jarl acted.

Sten-Hermann Schmidt
Vice president

---

a cancer patient and requesting that carcinoid patients not attempt to contact her. One day not so long ago when I was finishing up this book, the mailman delivered one of the CARPA bulletins J sent from Sweden. When I opened it, the first thing my eye fell on was the one-page obituary of J. I was in my studio at the time and stood watching two birds pecking in the grass in our back yard. J had told me many things about his cancer. He was a survivor of eighteen years who had served as a model to us all, a personal ray of hope. Only a few months earlier he had travelled to the USA to visit other patients and consult Doctor W, a carcinoid specialist, in New York, and Doctor W's wife M, a specialist in diet for cancer patients. He reported on that occasion that he'd enjoyed immensely a huge beef steak he'd consumed in the company of the Ws. As always, he'd seemed upbeat about recounting his travels and positive about cancer treatment. But he hadn't revealed that his own case had gone into a downward spiral. I would like to have given him my encouragement; I would like to have said goodbye. I watched the birds hopping about on the lawn, and after a while I sat on a chair and stared at the carpet, not knowing what I should think.

-Will you go away?

-No, dear boy, cancer does *not* go away.

-People become stable—I have become stable. Treatments succeed; remissions occur. With good care, good luck, and great faith, some patients are cured.

-But we do not go away.

-You come back?

-We were always there, and we will continue always to be there. We *are*. But not with malice or dark intent. Listen to your heart beat. Always there. Conceive an equation. Learn to see cancer that way. Learn *something*, for heaven's sake.

-So, you're always waiting.

-OK. Have it your way. We wait for you to weaken, for your immune system to go down.

-Then you pounce!

-Really, how dramatic! How soap opera sensational!

-You are monstrous. You lurk around corners, you pounce on victims like a jaguar in the night. You should be smashed out of existence.

-This is a dialogue, remember. But you're calling names again.

-I cannot be objective and liberal and indifferent about this. I'm dying because of you, you *aberrant* cells, you plague, you—

-And learning things about yourself.

-Crap.

-Here's something else you can learn: your fits of pique show that you know we're right. They show your inner weakness and reveal your alarm. They betray the fact that you know we speak the truth.

-Go to hell.

-As you will.

# Cam Shafts,
# Drive Trains, CV Boots

*It is incident to physicians beyond all other men to
mistake subsequence for consequence.*

—Samuel Johnson

In my years of suffering from and dealing with cancer I have
had the immense good fortune to encounter capable and
helpful physicians. For those of us with serious diseases, the
doctors who attend to our illnesses and advise us on courses
of treatment become, in a very real sense, the key people in
our lives, so it's important that they be many things, including sympathetic, intelligent, responsive, skillful, and caring.

What is a good physician? The answer varies with the circumstances. A good family doctor is someone who listens well
when you tell your initial "story"; someone who gauges accurately the dimensions of your concern; someone with strong
and reliable intuitions about you and about the entire spectrum of ailments; someone who works in a responsive network of family doctors and specialists and recommends you to
the best diagnosticians available. In this regard, my family
physician, M, a former student from my teaching days, was a
paragon in his occupation: after hearing about my visit to the

emergency ward and the "pink lady" treatment I received there, he put me on to the very best gastrointestinal man in our city. I was diagnosed correctly for a rare disease in a very brief time at an early stage of the ailment. (Since I've been in contact through e-mail with other carcinoid patients, I have discovered that many were mis-diagnosed for some time, critical months and years, in several cases.)

A commendable specialist has some additional qualities to those possessed by the capable family physician. Like the latter, the specialist must also be an effective listener, but here experience is important, experience with the whole gamut of ailments related to an area of specialization. Intelligence, too, is critical. Doctor MF, who diagnosed my cancer, represents for me the definition of this quality: a quick mind, an open mind, a discerning mind. In addition, Doctor MF is a superb technician; able to perform, for example, the painful and tricky colonoscopy procedure with maximum results. For adept hands and an able mind, patients must be ever grateful.

The specialist in nuclear medicine, Doctor WL, who first listened to M's queries about the radio-isotope procedure that we set in motion two years after I was diagnosed, was another gifted physician. I sensed from our first meeting that he was a brilliant man: he possessed an unusual combination of quickness of mind and lightness of character. But he was also extremely open to experiment and terrifically perceptive about how to go about the unusual procedure we attempted. A man of my own age, he was filled with youthful enthusiasm and vigorous determination, just the sort of person to whom you'd entrust your ailing body. His good humour and sensible advice were also welcome.

The oncologists who've handled my case, Doctors KK, WD, and AM, have all impressed me with their knowledge of cancer's operations and with their openness to discuss the progress of my disease and the treatments that might best be employed in dealing with it. Though overworked and sometimes visibly affected by the difficulties of practising in oncology (I don't know how these people hold up day to day with death so present and imminent in their routines), they have almost always offered me sensible advice about my disease; furthermore, they have been open with me about my status and prospects, and willing to cooperate with any suggestions I've dared to venture.

Was it one of the prophets who said, "Physician, heal thyself"? A good physician is one who knows his or her own limitations as well as those of the patients. Given the general reverence in which physicians are held in our culture, it must at times be difficult for doctors not to take themselves too seriously. (The converse can also be said: doctors may balk at being questioned or second-guessed by patients.) Whatever the case, here is a useful way to consider any doctor's contribution to our health: encouraging the patient to see herself as a partner in the undertaking, the physician engages the patient's creative energies in the task of healing, ever mindful of the key premise of a medical education: above all, do no harm.

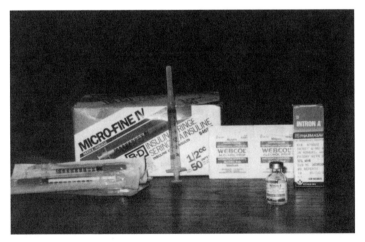

It may seem obvious, but I need to remind myself sometimes of a critical notion. Though specialists in oncology (or in any other area of medicine) know the diseases they're treating from extensive experience with many patients and wide reading about a host of ailments, none—or nearly none of them—actually have these diseases themselves. It takes me a moment to grasp the full implications of this obvious proposition. When I report to them that I feel X, my physicians may nod sagely and comprehend what I am telling them, but they do not themselves feel what I feel; they do not feel X. I want to believe—every patient does—that my physicians do feel X (and on other days Y and Z). BUT. My physicians, no matter how experienced with cancers, no matter how sensitive to my feelings and fears, do not know the sensations, pains, and anxieties of having this disease in their bodies. What the disease actually feels like. Further, most of them have never themselves experienced a CT scan, or a gastroscopy, or a colonoscopy, or a biopsy. Maybe they've never even had bloodwork, that nauseating arm-poking with a needle, about which every nurse who performs it confides to me, "I couldn't stand it myself." In short, my physicians' knowledge of what I'm suffering is all exterior. They know how cancer operates from the prospect of an outsider, but not what it feels like from the inside out, as I do.

Most of us who drive cars have what can be termed "dashboard knowledge" of the internal combustion engine and how it functions along with a transmission to power our vehicles. We push the levers and turn the knobs on the dashboard and the whole thing works. Miraculous! But we do not understand very well at all about valves, about cam shafts, about Bendix gears, about CV boots, carburetors, drive trains, and so on. If we've seen a spark plug outside of an engine, we do not know how it functions, much less how to "gap" one, or clean it. How much more complex the human organism—and mysterious and mystifying to patients and physicians alike!

In many respects doctors know more about the human body than we do, in the same way mechanics know more about the functioning of cars than does the average person. But since doctors are dealing with an organism, not a machine, their knowledge is circumscribed by the vast complexities of each and every human body: though similar, no one cancer case exactly parallels another. Not to mention the way the less tangible aspects of our beings—mind, spirit, soul, whatever we choose to call these things—affect the functioning of this complex organism in both positive and negative ways.

Physicians are our guides to better health, but no physician working alone can cure us. Other factors are equally significant. It's widely thought, for example, that any organism under siege from an infection responds by undertaking a series of creative adaptations to combat the trauma. So healing occurs for an array of complex reasons, including the body's adaptive strategies, good fortune, and a patient's strong disposition to be cured. In this latter regard, it's important to keep in mind something that Bernie Siegel says in one of his books. According to him, only about a third of patients who visit him seem prepared to take up the issue with cancer. (The remainder fall into two categories—those who were looking for a reason to die, and who accept cancer as the agent to fill that role; and those who seem to say to physicians, "You're the expert, not me, so I'm not going to do anything to promote my recovery—cure me.")

It's important to keep in mind, too, that medical knowledge and practice vary from place to place as well as from era to era; and that, in consequence, physicians have been educated and trained somewhere by someone at some time. The knowledge they have has been passed on to them by older physicians, people with wisdom and experience, yes, but also with prejudices and biases and—perhaps—outdated or inadequate information. Physicians *do* have biases. I was astonished to learn in this respect that European physicians and those practising in the United States often take different approaches when treating cancers. In Europe, carcinoid cancer is generally treated more aggressively than in the United States. European physicians recommend resection of the primary tumour and an aggressive course of interferon; American physicians tend to disregard primary tumours and to recommend the use of somatostatin analogues (octreotide), drugs that manage symptoms. As a patient you may never discover that two quite divergent approaches exist in combatting your disease; if you do, you can become confused by this divergence of views (each held passionately by its adherents) and may be in a quandary as to which set of procedures to follow. There's no simple solution. Without engaging in the debate, a useful tip might be the following: discover, if you can, how many patients have been treated by the oncologist you are seeing (or the one being relied on for advice and instruction); the wider the oncologist's experience of the disease, the larger the "pool" of patients treated, and the longer your physician has been dealing with your particular ailment, the more likely you are to receive advice with long-term prospects for success.

Recovery may be further complicated by the fact that not all decisions regarding patient care are directly in the hands of doctors in the way patients usually assume. Doctors work at hospitals and are frequently enmeshed in institutional politics, and this means shortages of funds to pursue the newest (and often most expensive) treatments; conflicts with other doctors over "territory"; and institutional policies that bind the hands of doctors for a host of reasons, not all of which are sensible, or even rational. There must repeatedly be occasions when physicians wish to pursue a course of treatment but cannot for reasons largely having nothing to do with the physician's knowledge or disposition to a patient's case. In circumstances where patients pay for consultations and treatments, physicians must also frequently feel hamstrung by monetary considerations.

Everyone seems to know this old saw: "What's the difference between God and a doctor?" Answer: "God doesn't think he's a doctor." Whether or not this snide riposte is accurate to the personalities of most physicians, the jest reminds us of something very important: we need physicians; they are our most powerful allies in the journey we are embarked upon. We have to work with them, but we must also recognize that their good humour, their intelligence, their sane judgement, their good intentions may not be enough to bring us to the recovery we so keenly desire. We accept that we may not be able to miraculously cure ourselves; neither may they.

-You don't want to keep talking, dear boy?

-If I do, if I take your points seriously, then I acknowledge you, I grant you legitimacy and credibility. I want to kill you, not give you life.

-You would rather sulk and blame.

-I would rather be healthy.

-Pooh. You have no idea what that means. Right now you eat three meals every day, you play sports, you take the occasional glass of wine, you have sex, you go on long walks, you write books, you play with your child, you sleep well.

-Reasonably well. Never through the night. My guts roil and boil. I sweat. I wake with a dry mouth and with pounding headaches. I suffer diarrhea, my face and chest flush from the hormones overloading my body, hormones you produce as by-products: serotonin and the like. I have to check my bowel movements, peer into the toilet in order to monitor what's going on inside me. It's demeaning, undignified, and disgusting. As for sports, I perform them at a diminished level. I'm half the man I once was because the drug I take weakens me.

-This is carping. Poor baby.

-Not to mention psychological health.

-See a psychiatrist, a psychologist. Consult the Buddha. Meditate. Fall back on resources you never even knew were at your disposal. But do not carp about your psychic health to us! We're dying!

-*You're dying!* This is ridiculous.

-Is it? Every day you inject a powerful drug whose purpose is to destroy mutated cells. You have taken radiation treatments to wipe us out—annihilate us! You eat vitamin C because it's an anti-cancer agent; you drink green tea with polyphenols that attack us; you consume broccoli sprouts for the sulphorophane that weakens us so the antioxidants can more easily destroy us. You are contemplating surgery on your bowel and a treatment called embolization, which blocks the blood to our cells and kills us. So you have declared war on us, all-out war; and yet we are supposed to blithely listen to you complaining about your precious health—diminished sexual capacity. Give over!

-You said earlier that you were; that you had to flourish. Ditto from this side.

-So you send in your assassins.

-Now who's calling names?

# Waiting Room

*The secret of the care of the patient is in caring for the patient.*

—Francis Peabody

Sometimes the word "clinic" refers to the building where patients meet with a physician, as in Downtown Clinic. *Clinic* also has a more refined meaning in medical circles: an occasion when doctors practising a particular kind of medicine meet with patients suffering from common ailments. Hence, a cancer clinic. The shift in meaning is perhaps less important than what the word "clinic" has come to mean for most patients.

Clinics are meant to be opportunities for patients to discuss with physicians both their personal condition and the status of the treatments they are undergoing. The clinic is supposed to be informative and helpful. Maybe an obstetrics clinic is a place where upbeat physicians meet with happy, expectant mothers to discuss their well-being and the progress of their foetus's development. Perhaps, I like to imagine, nurses bustle about briskly carrying files about new life; and laughter rings out along the corridors from time to time.

Oncology clinics are not like this.

In general medical practice these days, patients should understand, they are usually the fourth most important group of people in a clinic setting. First there are the doctors, the high priests of medicine; then come the nurses, the physicians' attendants; then the reception/processing cadre, whom we first meet and generally encounter on the telephone and behind raised counters; and finally, the patients. You know where you stand after your first clinic experience when the receptionist takes your name upon your arrival and tells you one thing and one thing only, "Please take a seat." This is the beginning of The Wait. After some time, a half hour in most cases, on rare occasions as little as fifteen minutes, but sometimes as much as an hour and a half, your name is called and you are directed from the large waiting room to the small, the cubicle where the examination and consultation take place. Here you wait another ten or fifteen minutes. (I cannot help thinking that in this intervening period my attending physician is frantically flipping through my file, trying to remember desperately who I am and what I was told during the last visit.)

Doctors, of course, are busy. So are nurses. Still, someone could tell you from the outset a few simple details regarding your visit: how long the wait in the exterior waiting room is expected to be, for instance. But the standard practice is to tell patients as little as necessary. This is the definition of "paternalistic attitude," and the clinic, as it is run these days, specializes in it. When the nurse takes you down to the consultation cubicle she often again says nothing, or merely, "Wait here." If you are needing bloodwork after your consultation, a nurse will tell you, "Go to the end of the hall and tell them you need bloodwork." *Them?* You stumble off in that direction, feeling helpless and out of control. The first time this happened to me, I was surprised when I located *them* to be bluntly told, "Roll up your sleeve." Then the needle was stuck in my vein. Queasy following the consultation with my physician, I passed out.

Before this turns into a rant, let me say there's no malice

here, as far as I can tell. Nurses are busy and stressed out; they're called upon to perform too many tasks, to be too many things to too many people: assistants to doctors, bookkeepers to the hospital, guides to patients. Physicians are overburdened with patients and paperwork. Receptionists face a bank of ringing phones and blinking computer screens. All that aside, it seems to me as if health care workers forget what's actually going on in a cancer clinic: ailing people, many frightened to the cores of their beings, are about to consult with physicians about the single most important aspect of their lives—their continued existence. Often—almost always—they are in a fragile state, physically and mentally. Many are just managing to hold themselves together. Probably the last thing they need at such times is to be pushed about from place to place like so much meat and told almost nothing about what is about to happen to them, or how long they will be expected to wait before it happens.

In consequence, it can sometimes be bewildering to be a patient; on occasion it can be downright humiliating.

Physicians and nurses, overworked as they are, sometimes forget certain basic givens of patient care. The first of these is that the patient is the person being attended to. Yet far too often, we patients receive the impression that our appointments, our tests, and so on, are being arranged and orchestrated to suit the needs of the physician attending us or the schedules of the institution where we are being treated. We are presented with a statement of a *fait accompli*. A paternalistic assumption operates here that can be quite off-putting. I'm sometimes tempted to ask, "Who's the patient here?" To which the answer must inevitably be: the person being asked to show the most patience.

Secondly, there is this fact of life to consider. Most of us diagnosed as adults have enjoyed a considerable measure of control over our existences. As foremen in shops, as professionals, or teachers, or secretaries in large organizations, as operators of small businesses—whatever—we daily make decisions, are consulted for opinions, and work independently at complex tasks. Then something dramatic imposes itself into our lives. We experience a traumatic injury; or we suffer a serious ailment; or we are diagnosed with a disease. We feel not only that our bodies have betrayed us—at the very least let us down—but also that our lives to a large extent are spinning out of control. Things are happening to us and we are more or less powerless to alter the situation. Treatments, remedies, therapies may be available; but much of what little can be done to improve the situation is in the hands of other people.

That's a frightening feeling, one that takes time to adapt to. Physicians and nurses could help us with this issue, but almost always they make it worse. They exacerbate the situation by assuming total control of our treatments as well as of our routines in the clinic. They tell us only oddments about our disease and about where we fall on the spectrum from incidence to mortality; they order us about with minimum explanation; they schedule procedures after slight or no consultation with patients. The end result is that patients entering clinics feel doubly out of control: helpless to alter the course of their ailment, they find themselves shunted about seemingly at the whim of the very clinic workers who should be tempering their distress. It's doubly demeaning. So if some patients' sense of this diminishment occasionally flares into resentment against workers in the clinic, it should not come as a surprise.

In the past few years I've developed a number of strategies to deal with clinic waiting. It doesn't hurt, I've discovered, to call ahead on the day of your appointment—a half hour ahead, say—to find out whether the doctor is physically present at the clinic. If she is, it's also useful to ask, "Are the appointments on schedule?" If not, "How long is the wait—how far is the physician behind schedule?" No one will volunteer this information, but if you ask, you can often find out. This can at least minimize the wait of an hour and a half when the doctor has been held up during "rounds" (typically scheduled in the mornings), or by some procedure that she is attending (another patient's surgery, say).

In an oncology clinic there is a kind of hush over the

corridors. The outer waiting room is peopled by patients in varying states of distress. The occasional person looks truly frightened. Someone else is grey and drawn in appearance; things are not going well. At the clinic I attend there are often women in the waiting room, victims of breast cancer. They often speak with fellow sufferers; perhaps they are in support groups together or have encountered each other in this setting before. Maybe women are just more open than men about ailments. Men tend to sit quietly with their hands on the arms of the chairs, breathing through their mouths and waiting stoically to see the doctor. We've been trained to tough it out, suffer in silence, and we do. Very few people in clinics read. There was a television in the waiting room at one time. No one watched it. A year or two ago, it disappeared. In any case, the women sitting across or next to me are remarkably candid with each other. They say things like this: "I was doing well after the surgery, but then it moved into my lungs and we're going through all of it again." Or, "My weight is down twenty pounds; I can't keep it up; it's a sure sign things are going downhill, but they think the chemo might help." Or, "You remember Julie, she went fast." Nods, murmurs. I'm fascinated by these exchanges, but repelled by them as well. They shake me up: talk of things going badly, of death, unnerves us all, but in these circumstances, when one is about to consult a physician about one's condition, the upset can cut deep. I feel nauseous. Sometimes when I'm called to see my physician, I rise from my seat shaking and with my stomach in a knot. I understand why many patients bring their spouses or a friend with them: having someone close to you to talk with during The Wait distracts you from bleak thoughts and buffers the distress.

Often the people who accompany patients go into the consultation room with them. This, too, is a commendable strategy. Patients are upset when they attend a clinic, and a second set of ears can be useful in recalling what the physician said. Even if that is not the case, all of us hear selectively, and a day, a week, a month later it's sometimes difficult to recall exactly

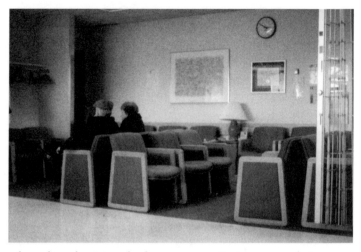

what the physician had to report. Patients, or their team members, can jot down a few notes during the consultation with the physician, so that at a later date the patient has reliable details to conjure with, rather than blurry impressions and faded memories. While this may trouble some physicians, most are open to the idea and welcome it.

I have also discovered that you have to work at the consultation itself. Whether from delicacy about our feelings as victims of disease, or by nature and training, or from overwork, doctors typically do not tell patients very much. They may say, "You're doing well," or something noncommittal of that kind. You need to press them for specifics, to ask, "What were the numbers on that last blood count?" or "Can you tell me what the Chromogranin level is in a healthy person?" It took me almost a year to ask Doctor KK about the size of the tumours in my liver. I'd thought they were numerous and fairly large—golfball size, perhaps. It turned out they were smaller and far less numerous than I'd imagined. All to my immense relief. On another occasion I was read the radiology report from my most recent CT scan: the tumours, it was reported, had grown a little. I dared to ask, "How is that measured?" and then, when my physician looked at me oddly, I persisted, asking, "Can I see the two most recent pictures for myself?" When the negatives were placed in the viewing device, the physician measured each set of tumours with a pair of calipers. Try as we might, neither of us could detect any change from the earlier set of negatives to the later. "Well," my physician said, "maybe there really hasn't been any change." I went home relieved, rather than upset, which I would have been had I not pressed for more information.

My point here is not to criticize the physicians attending me or to undermine the medical procedures that have been performed on me. Everyone I've encountered, I am convinced, is doing their best. Receptionists, nurses, and physicians alike have been friendly and helpful. My point is that if you don't ask, if you allow yourself to be cowed by the clinic, you may receive faulty information or not enough information, and you may leave the clinic upset or frightened when you need not be. Oncology is not a happy business. We all get depressed at times. We all have our down periods. But we need not have more of them than necessary, and imaginings can often be worse than the genuine knowledge. Perhaps it's in my makeup to want to hear the worst and deal with it. That can be painful, I admit. But I'd rather that than passively accept whatever someone else—even a well-meaning physician—decides I am allowed to hear. Every patient leaves every clinic a little shaken. Even when the news is good. That I accept. I know, too, that tomorrow is another day, and the more information I'm armed with, the better able I will be to continue the fray.

-So, you will not go away?

-We simply exist. An inexorable fact. That point has been made already.

-But if you will not go away by your own choosing, then I can use what I have learned to combat you.

-Believe what you will.

-I believe that I am stronger now and can fight you off. This dialogue—an exercise that seemed futile when we began, and still does sometimes—this dialogue has opened my eyes. I understand a little better than I did before.

-See?

-Piss off. I'm saying that with knowledge and with insight, as well as with drugs and treatments and surgeries, I can fight you off.

-Do what you will.

-You're becoming tight-lipped. You know I'm right. Your silence betrays it.

-Does it?

-You said so earlier—you said that silence and rancour show fear, and now it's back on you with that one, *dear boy.*

-Do what you can. Take whatever course you must.

-I can defeat you, then? You grant that?

-*Defeat?*

-Transcend.

-Think what you must.

# Hot and Sour Soup,
# Shrimp Rolls, Football

*It's what you have to do with every disease: act like
you don't have it and keep on going.*
—Angelo Dundee on Muhammad Ali's
"pugilist's syndrome"

Throughout most of the year 1995 I was on the biological
modification drug Alpha-Interferon 2b, which I injected subcutaneously, like a diabetes patient, every day. It was supposed
to support my immune system, providing a catalyst to the
killer-T cells at work in my blood system, as in everyone's,
destroying cancer cells and other infected cells in the body. At
first I reacted to the interferon, as my physicians had all
advised I would, with symptoms of fever: sweating,
headaches, weakness, and some flushing. They had recommended I inject the drug before retiring for the day so as to
sleep through these effects, and that was good advice. After a
week or ten days, the symptoms subsided.

That year saw me become familiar with certain routines:
every three months or so I went in to the hospital for a CT
scan. Radiologists studied these scans and after a time reported good news: the primary tumour in the mid-section of my

gut and the metastases in the liver did not show evidence of growth. Just before each CT scan I had samples of blood taken from the veins in my arms and these samples were sent to the Mayo Clinic in Minnesota, where they were tested for Chromogranin A, a protein indicator that according to Doctor KO provided a reliable "marker" of the hormone activity in my system, and hence, the cancer activity. I also delivered to the Oncology Department at the Saint Boniface Hospital every three months a twenty-four-hour urine sample, which was used to ascertain levels of 5HIAA (more hormones and related chemicals in the body), and a second marker of biochemical activity proceeding from the cancer tumours. Over the following months my physicians assured me that the interferon was having the desired effect: the level of Chromogranin in my system dropped sharply, and a similar drop in levels of 5HIAA occurred.

At the same time I corresponded with my e-mail friends, learning how they were doing and what treatments were available for sufferers of carcinoid cancer. From time to time I talked with KT, who had arranged the visit of Doctor KO to Winnipeg. At one point I told KT I was restless with the way my treatment was proceeding: Doctor KO had recommended an aggressive course of treatment, including surgery, but Doctor KK seemed content tracking CT results and the numbers coming back from the Chromogranin A and 5HIAA samples. KT said, "There's an oncologist in Saskatoon who seems really interested in what you've got—why don't you call him, and if you feel like pursuing it, go visit him." KT was always offering this kind of down-to-earth advice.

Doctor AM turned out not just to be interested in the carcinoid phenomenon as I engaged it, but to be a truly genuine and warm human being. Talking with him on the phone, I felt the same comfort as when I discussed my case with my family physician, M. He told me about some trials being done in the Nuclear Medicine Department at the University of Alberta in Edmonton. "Get in touch with Doctor MC," he told me. And he gave me a telephone number.

At the University of Alberta, one of Doctor MC's assistants explained, they were trying a "smart bomb" approach to radiating certain cancers, including carcinoids. They had learned that cancer cells with certain "profiles" attracted to their surfaces certain chemical compounds. If they mixed these latter with radioactive matter, the radioactive materials bound themselves to the surfaces of the cancer cells and in this way tumour cells could be attacked from within the body rather than blasting them from the outside, as in conventional radiation therapy. It was genetic engineering of sorts, activating the body's receptor system to complement its normal humoral response to intrusions. In any case, to my layman's ears this is what the research doctor in Edmonton seemed to be telling me. She referred to the solution they used as radioactive isotopes and called the chemical that attacked the cancer cells I131 and the overall treatment MIBG. It sounded cutting edge and intriguing.

According to the doctor on the phone in Edmonton, they had had some good and some promising results from MIBG treatments, though the sample they had worked with (forty patients) was not large. (One patient had been cured, several others had seen dramatic tumour shrinkage.) They were willing to run me through the treatment, but it took almost two weeks: a preliminary run, using a weakened form of I131, was done to ascertain if there was sufficient "take-up" by the tumours; this might take four days or more to determine; after the actual treatment, which lasted one afternoon, the patient was required to be in isolation for three days to forestall radioactive contamination.

When I talked about this with M and showed him the page of graphs, statistics, and results the research doctor in Edmonton had faxed to me, he said, "What a great idea. Any procedure that allows you to avoid the intrusions of surgery should be tried." I explained that the treatment in Edmonton involved ten days or more away from home. He said, "Hang on a moment, I'm going to make a call." I was sitting across from him in his office on a Friday afternoon, when he should have been heading out the door to his wife. This response was typical M. Once when I'd expressed the concern that the physicians at the Saint Boniface Hospital might not have had a lot of experience doing embolizations, he picked up the phone as we were speaking and called a radiologist friend at Mount Sinai Hospital in Toronto. "One," M said when he put down the phone, "SB has every confidence in the radiologists at the Saint Boniface. Two, he'd be happy to set you up for an embolization in Toronto at any time." Unless you have been a patient with a life-threatening disease, it is difficult to appreciate how much these telephone calls that offer an immediate solution mean. There are options; there are alternatives; the medical system can be put in motion for your benefit. These things allay the deep-seated fear and helplessness in the face of the medical complex that all patients feel.

It seemed only a week later that I was in the cramped office of Doctor WL, head of the Nuclear Medicine Department at the Saint Boniface. A trim, greying man, Doctor WL's eyes sparkled with life and enthusiasm as he went over the steps of the MIBG treatment. Although he had never done one before, Doctor WL was eager to try radio-isotope therapy and confident that the facilities at the hospital were up to the treatment. He'd spoken at length with Doctor MC in Edmonton. "Only," he told me, "the maintenance department here is renovating the wing where we have our isolation unit, so we may have to wait a month or so."

In my naivete I didn't realize that he had given me a very optimistic time-line.

About five months later I went in for the preliminary scan, a process involving a small injection of I131 and a two-hour period under radiation cameras poised about one and half inches above my torso. ("Don't move!" cautioned the nurse.) I was apprehensive about this initial step. If there was not sufficient take-up of substance by the cell receptors, the procedure was off. And I was hopeful that this non-intrusive approach to the tumours might save me the pain and inconvenience of surgery. A week or so later Doctor KK told me over the phone, "You had good take-up on the MIBG. The tumours in your liver lit up like a Christmas tree."

A CT scan was done the day before the MIBG treatment—to provide a benchmark of the tumour development just prior to the procedure.

Here I faced a difficult moment. My son was four years old. I'd told him as much as a year earlier that I had cancer. What was I to tell him about this procedure? The physician who had done a preliminary hepatic angiogram on me said that there was a slim possibility of something going wrong. And I knew that every day of the week patients went into hospitals and did not come out. I did not want to alarm A, but neither did I wish to disappear from his life—what would he think in later years? A genuine dilemma. I was dropping him off at his mother's the morning of the procedure. I kneeled down beside him and hoisted him onto my knee. "There's something serious I must say," I began; "sometimes dads go into hospitals and don't come back. There's really no chance this will be case this time, but I wanted to tell you that and that I love you." My heart was pounding; I was holding his hand in mine. A's a redhead, like his mother—thick hair that sticks out every which way on the crown of his skull. "Me too," he said, and then in a moment, "it'll be all right, Dad." He patted my hand and jumped down off my knee and ran into his mother's house.

There was considerable bustle at the Saint Boniface the afternoon Doctor WL did the I131 treatment. It was a Friday in autumn. We were in the isolation room. I sat across from Doctor WL at a small wooden table, the sleeve of one arm rolled high. A nurse set an intravenous going and then another brought in what looked like a test tube filled with thin mercury. After some fiddling with this tube—it was placed in a kind of recessed glass case, open at both ends, and then the intravenous tubing was attached to it—the liquid was pushed into my arm by a pump attached at the far end of the tube. Doctors and nurses poked their heads into the room from time to time, nodding and smiling. Apparently I was a minor celebrity, the guy who in a few hours would be so radioactive that the room would be sealed on the first night.

In a half hour or so all the liquid was out of the tube and inside my body. Doctor WL performed a few simple tests on me—stethoscope to the heart, blood pressure scarf. Then he asked me how I felt. A little woozy but otherwise fine. He told me he'd be back to see me periodically over the next few days, and then he packed up his equipment and left. A nurse took away the table on which the equipment had been sitting. The door to the room was closed on its rubber seal.

There was a tiny television in the room. I'd brought some books. K had arrived just before Doctor WL departed, bringing bottled water and A. They were not allowed into the room, but stood behind a strap of yellow tape at the door, twenty feet between us, waving. When they left, I called out, "Bye, A," and he called back, "Bye, bye, Radioactive Man." He was chuckling. One of the characters on a television show he watched was called this.

That was a long three days. It was October. I watched American football on the microscopic television set. I read a novel. I picked at the hospital food a nurse slipped into the room, her smocked arm visible to the elbow as she positioned the tray and then withdrew hurriedly. I meditated; I fell asleep at about ten o'clock; at about eleven a nurse came noisily into the room and woke me up to ask me if I needed a sleeping pill; well, yes, I did then!

The next morning a nurse told me the door could be opened for visitors. A former student of mine from my days of teaching at a private school, and now a resident in Nephrology, stopped by to visit. He sat on the edge of the bed. "Doctor Tefs," he said, recalling the tone he'd used as a teenager. "Doctor CR," I said, trying out the sound of that, "aren't you afraid of the radiation?" He waved away this concern. "A lot of foolishness," he said. We joked about hospitals and the medical profession and about school days. Like Doctor WL, his face was alight with enthusiasm for his work. "I read your novels," he told me. "My wife, too."

In the early afternoon married friends, M and J, arrived with a steak and fries, which they placed just inside the door. We joked about radiation contamination. My friend M put his foot over the yellow tape and then mocked a sudden heart attack before withdrawing his foot. I told them I was feeling fine. They stood in the doorway and said, "We're going home to rake leaves." I'd looked out the one tiny window earlier: a bright but crisp fall day, a north wind swirling leaves up in the park across the road. We lived in a neighbourhood where it was not uncommon to fill fifty or a hundred plastic bags with leaves every autumn; it was an activity K and A and I did together, and that would have been fun. Later a second ex-student came in to visit. "Doctor Tefs," she said, "I was surprised to hear that you were here." "Doctor JC," I responded, "you look very tired." "Residency," she said, "I'm at the end of a fourteen-hour shift." Some hours later K and A arrived with my favourite oriental foods, a hot and sour soup and shrimp rolls, from an oriental restaurant we frequented.

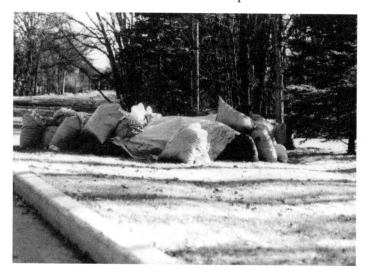

Doctor WL appeared shortly afterward with a bright smile on his face and a Geiger counter in one hand. He did some readings near the door and then next to my body. "Not bad,"

he reported, "not bad at all. At this rate the levels should fall enough so we can release you Monday morning." He checked my chest again. "How's the food?" he asked as he left. Possibly he smelled the non-institutional goodies that had been brought in.

That night I felt nauseous. I did not fall asleep until after eleven and awoke again at about one. I pictured the chemicals that had been introduced into my body making their way to the tumour in my gut and those in my liver, attacking the cancer cells and destroying them. I was not concerned that the powerful chemicals would find their way to other parts of my body and damage them; I was not afraid that they would impair my liver function; I was not apprehensive about other side effects. Maybe I should have been. Because he seemed to be a very smart man and a very competent one, I trusted Doctor WL implicitly, and he had told me that the odds of anything bad occurring from this treatment were one hundred to one. I rested easily and tried to pass the long hours in the tiny square room where everything that was not made of metal had been covered carefully with plastic. I had brought my meditation candle with me and I sat concentrating on the flickering flame for long stretches of time. I wondered about the fire regulations—would that tiny bit of smoke set off the alarms?

Sunday. Football, football, football. I dozed. I picked at the food the nurses brought in. I talked with K on the phone in the isolation room. On Sunday afternoon one of my sisters came to the door. Then my mother. Then my other sister with her husband. Cheery waves from the hallway. Mid-afternoon on Sunday Doctor WL visited again, and after checking his Geiger counter said I could go home first thing on Monday. That night I slept soundly. On Monday morning I was packed and ready to go at 9:00 AM.

The follow-up CT scan that was performed three months after the 1131 treatment, the three months giving the radio-isotope ample time to work on the cancer cells, showed no change from the previous scan. When I consulted with him,

Doctor KK said, "These things take time." At the outset of the radio-isotope procedure I had dared to hope that the tumours in my liver would shrink dramatically (in Edmonton one patient undergoing the treatment had been "cured"—the tumours had disappeared). When I spoke with him on the phone, M said, "It may be six months or more before we see the results of this treatment." And in a follow-up meeting, Doctor WL said, "There was tremendous take-up. I think that if we don't see actual tumour shrinkage, we'll see the tumours stabilize over the long stretch."

I went back to my writing and to playing hockey on Sunday mornings, Tuesday nights, and Friday afternoons. I shovelled snow, bought a giant Lego pirate ship for A at Christmas, drank the occasional glass of red wine, flew to Mexico with A and K for two weeks in the sun the following February. The CT scans that were done in April, in September, and in December of the following year showed no tumour growth. The subsequent five years have been the same—fifteen scans, no change. Sometimes no news *is* good news.

-The point is, if I cannot defeat you, I can live through you.

-Oh, do give over, dear boy.

-Yes, it does sound smug.

-Cancer is not intentionally malicious, you know? Malignant, but not malicious.

-I think I understand the answer to *Why me?*

-You're taking a lot on yourself. You were easier to stomach when you were going on about your precious bloody health and your precious bloody sex life. Kvetching.

-A friend who has a daughter with a brain tumour said to me recently: "You two are amazing; a model to us all."

-People say silly things.

-She was referring to the way we fight you off each day. She knows from the inside how this works: trips to the Mayo Clinic, desperate hours waiting for test results, tearful embraces in antiseptic corridors. Her daughter has a son of six years. If she dies, what will happen to him? My friend used the word "courageous."

-People do blather on.

-She meant we were an example to others, that our struggle made us models that others could look to in confronting their own trials in life.

-People are sentimental idiots who want to believe in goodness triumphing and in progress and improvement and growth.

-You said I had grown, *dear* boy.

-You're quite repugnant when you do that—throw back words in that way.

-You said that good things came from having cancer. Let me put it bluntly: I was blind to certain things: the needs of other people. Blind to their vulnerabilities, which I regarded as weakness. I was blind to compassion, and demanding of others, and hard on myself. I thought I had standards, but what my behaviours demonstrated was lack of forgiveness.

-You are becoming boring, you know? Your little speeches are so much loose tin rattling in the wind. Go away.

-As you will.

# Styrofoam
# and Swizzle Sticks

*You should blow out your candle to find yourself*
*more clearly.*

—Denis Diderot

Several months after I was diagnosed with carcinoid cancer, I was going over things with my family physician, M, in his office. "Do you think," I asked him, "I should see a psychiatrist?" He did not hesitate. "You seem to be doing well in that regard," he told me, "but it never hurts to talk these things through with a professional. So, sure, if you want to see somebody, I can recommend a man highly. You'll find him, I believe, to be sensible and down-to-earth."

M was right. Doctor FS worked out of his home, a rambling, multi-storey affair in one of the trendy areas of our city. His consulting office was located on the main floor off a waiting room that had once been the sitting room of the house. There was a pot of coffee on a small side table and Styrofoam cups and swizzle sticks. Inside the consulting room proper there were the usual professional accoutrements: filing cabinets, a few prints by local artists, book shelves, degrees in frames on the walls.

Doctor FS was a short man who told me he ran in the marathon when I noted he looked trim and fit. He had a notepad on one knee and was jotting down my particulars as we chatted: age, marital status, kind of cancer, general health, and so on. He wanted to know what drugs I was on—or had been taking prior to being diagnosed. I told him about some minor back pains I'd suffered after vigorous cycling on the ridgeways in England—and the naproxen I'd taken for it. Also about the migraine headaches I'd suffered some years earlier—only after playing hockey—and the Cafergot I'd taken for relief. I told him about my conversation with Doctor Y, the neurologist who had examined me back then.

I had asked Doctor Y, "What can I do about these headaches?"

He'd said, "Do you only get them after playing hockey?"

"Yes."

"Then stop playing hockey," Doctor Y told me. He and I had laughed about that at the time. Then he had prescribed the Cafergot.

Doctor FS and I laughed about the incident now. "Some remedies," he observed, "are easier than others."

We chatted about the sudden death of my father, which had occurred about fifteen months before I was diagnosed; and the birth of my son, which had occurred some fifteen months prior to that. I'd been dismissed from my job in there, too, and separated from my former wife in the same period. "Lots of changes," Doctor FS said. I told him about Carl Simonton's observations regarding stress in his book, *Getting Well Again*. Simonton says that most people who contract cancer have had a dramatic event occur in their lives within eighteen months of being diagnosed (sometimes more than one such dramatic event). His conclusion seems to be this: cancer is present in all of us all of the time, the mutating aberrant cells that constitute "cancer," in any case; when our bodies weaken under stress (the death of a loved one qualifies highly, but so does the birth of a child, or a wedding), the cancer has an opportunity to come to the fore, and can, if we are not alert, invade our bodies. It's a sensible proposition: in times of stress our immune systems can falter, opening us up to the invasion of a latent disease. Doctor FS agreed that this made sense.

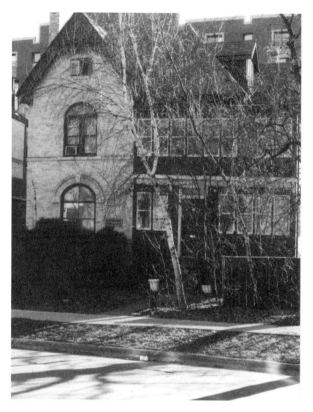

He asked me about my relationship with K. I told him we were happy and sketched for him our plans for travelling in Europe the coming summer, as well as our intention of adding a screened room to our house, to include a hot tub, projects that we were both enthusiastic about. He asked me how K was doing, and I assured him that she was coping well. We talked about A and about the teaching I was doing at the university. At the conclusion of our hour, we shook hands and

Doctor FS told me to make a follow-up appointment to see him in three months.

I left feeling somewhat let down. Having read Carl Simonton's uplifting book, I was expecting, I guess, to have Doctor FS probe deeply into the state of my psyche and then recommend a course of purposeful activities, including a spectrum of goals for me to achieve, or some such thing. Instead our talk had been laid back, laconic, low-key. I had done a lot of the talking, but did not feel particularly relieved or refreshed by what we'd accomplished in our session. That night I told K about these misgivings. "Maybe you want too much," she said. She reminded me that in graduate school I'd done a lot of reading in psychoanalysis and perhaps had anticipated something "heavy" to occur with Doctor FS that was not going to happen, and perhaps should not. I was not, she pointed out, in crisis about my cancer, or generally a neurotic person. She quoted the line from a novel at me, about being abnormally normal, and we laughed at that. I was comforted in a way by her reassurances—but only in a way.

In three months I saw Doctor FS again. He'd competed in a marathon in one of the big American cities and had recorded a personal best time. He wanted to know how I was feeling. Good. He seemed especially interested to know how things were going with K. I sensed he was probing into the stability of our relationship, perhaps fearful that I might be left on my own at this delicate moment in my life, abandoned by someone who did not want to deal with *cancer*. He jotted notes and asked how K herself was doing. I reassured him on this score and then asked, "Should she see a psychiatrist?" He shook his head. "Not if she's doing all right and has not expressed the desire." We left it at that.

I returned in another three months. I always enjoyed our chats, but I did not feel that we were getting anywhere. Maybe we weren't supposed to. Maybe I was suffering the illusion that progress in this area—accomplishing something— would have a positive effect on the progress of my cancer. It's an equation that can tempt a victim of a serious disease:

improvement in psychological terms can seem to herald improvement in physical ways. We patients are prone to look for these signs, or portents. Probably Doctor FS knew this and did not want me to fabricate false hopes. These thoughts rattled around in my brain from time to time. Then one day I was talking with my sister S. "If you're not pleased with this line of therapy," she said, "why don't you see someone else?" She recommended a Doctor JS, a psychologist who had an office in a house on another trendy street in our city: specialty food shops, cafes, delis, fashion boutiques, health food stores.

Doctor JS was a bearded man who shook my hand warmly. He conducted me on a brief tour of the premises: waiting rooms, consulting rooms, in the basement a carpeted room with carpeted square modules and boxes of children's toys along one wall. "We do therapy to expose the wounded child," he said by way of explanation. I thought he meant *with* emotionally disturbed children. Upstairs we sat across from each other on matching leather chairs. Doctor JS had a notepad on his knee and he took down some particulars. "We're interested here," he told me, "in the lost child inside you." I shifted on my chair. Doctor JS sensed my discomfort, but went on, "We deal with a lot of Natives here, we hold group sessions where we try to open up to the damaged child within our adult selves, our inner child." I was beginning to get the picture: not children playing with toys, but adults playing with children's toys as a way of exploring the traumas of childhood, suppressed and locked hurtfully inside. "It's a rich area, the inner child," he continued, "emotionally speaking."

We looked at each other for some minutes. "Tell me about the death of your father," he said. In a few moments I sketched in the details: how my mother found my father in the bathroom, where he'd gone to urinate. He'd died instantly from a massive infarction. "How did you feel about him?" Doctor JS asked. "He was a wonderful man," I told Doctor JS. Because he had been. Doctor JS asked, "Was he a good father? Did he love you and your sisters as much as you loved him?" I sensed my eyes were blurring; I was trembling inside and out. I was suddenly overcome by powerful feelings of loss. We sat in silence for some time. "I think," Doctor JS said, "that you would really benefit from our inner child group sessions. We are starting a new one next week." We walked to the entrance together, and after I'd written a cheque, he pressed a brochure about the group sessions into my hand.

In the parking lot I sat in my car for some time, pondering what had occurred. The near emotional breakdown I'd experienced in the consulting room concerned me. I felt betrayed. I did not want to outright deny what Doctor JS had triggered in me: the muddle of emotions that were still fomenting inside me from my father's death and the birth of my son and the separation from my former wife and the diagnosis of cancer. At the same time, I felt used, perhaps manipulated is more accurate. (It might be said in his defense that provoking an intense response, as Doctor JS had done, breaks us down and is a short-cut way to break through to feelings long buried, but this method also produces shame, and not all patients are ready and willing to confront shame early in their therapy.) And I was not sure that delving into the damaged child inside me, however revealing that might be about the relationship I had had with my parents, would really address the issue most crucial to me at the time: the cancer in my intestines and liver.

Perhaps I made a wrong turning at this juncture. I did not return to visit Doctor JS again. Was I afraid of what might be uncovered in his damaged child group sessions? Probably. But more important, I thought then, and think now, I was uncomfortable with the "program" that Doctor JS seemed intent on foisting on me. That is something that occurs often, I suspect, in circumstances where people freshly diagnosed with a serious disease turn to whomever is available for help. We are quite vulnerable at these times—emotionally fragile, bewildered, physically exhausted. We turn to others in good faith, trusting they will treat us kindly and aid in combatting our ailment. Too often this does not occur. Seen in the best light, it might be simply a matter of divergent expectations. We patients expect, I think, to be seen as individual sufferers; we expect the consultants we seek out to listen to us and then to respond to our difficulties by proposing therapies tailored to our unique circumstances. Instead, I sense, many therapists want to fit us into their agenda, to have us become part of their remedial experimenting. What I am saying here should not be misunderstood. I do not think that psychologists and therapists are charlatans. I do not even believe that they willfully blind themselves to the needs of the people who seek them out. They are, though, at least sometimes, so intent on their program that they can overlook the fact that it is not suited to every patient equally.

At one point in the first year subsequent to diagnosis, K and I visited an herbalist. She talked with us for a while, then had us fill out forms that helped her build a profile of our habits and characters: typical foods eaten, alcohol consumption, a schedule of bowel movements, and so on. After reviewing this material, the herbalist told us what type each of us was: K was *adrenaline* and I was *thyroidal*. (It sounded a lot to me like the four humours of the medieval cosmology: sanguinary, choleric, melancholic, phlegmatic; not unuseful categories, admittedly, but possibly less helpful than more sophisticated diagnoses.) We were told we should cleanse our bodies by eating only a very restricted diet, and then subsequently recommended a course of dietary supplements and herbal remedies—on sale in her shop—that would stabilize and strengthen our physiognomies. We followed the herbalist's recommendations. Perhaps they helped us. I would not wish to denigrate the good work such people do. Often they may help us—to at least realize how important what we consume is to our general health. At the very least, they can do little harm. I am less concerned about that than the fact that patients are so often fitted into a program by the people they seek out to help them. Perhaps it can be no other way. Each therapist, to achieve successful results, has to buy into a doctrine, an overall way of seeing life, what might be called a "world view." When we seek their help, they conclude—without telling us—that we wish to buy into their world view, too. So it is certainly useful to be aware of this tendency in care-givers, to keep in mind the fact that a degree of wariness about the people we pay to help us can be a useful strategy; they may have other motives than our good health in mind as they treat us.

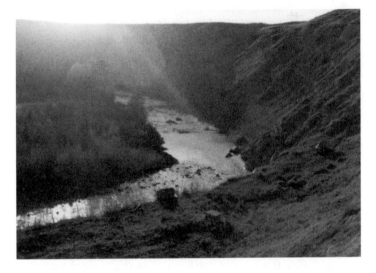

In the end, the experiment with the psychologist, Doctor JS, proved as ungratifying as that with the psychiatrist, Doctor FS. I admit I was looking for something in the line of regeneration. I had read Carl Simonton's *The Healing Journey* and had found his account of one patient's restorative pilgrimage very uplifting. Reid Henson had righted himself after a frightening diagnosis and had employed numerous strategies to help him become well again, including keeping a journal and seeking out a spiritual healer. I myself am not a religious person in any conventional sense, having abandoned during my college days the Lutheranism in which I was raised. I confess, though, to leanings in the spiritual direction: a belief in the goodness of people, a sense that there is more to life than the fundamentals of birth, procreation, and death. (I'm susceptible to Hamlet's quip: "There are more things in heaven and earth than are dreamt of in your philosophy.") In this regard I'd long felt a spiritual connection to a landscape in Alberta. Just where the foothills begin, about twenty miles west of Calgary, my former in-laws lived in a high and airy wooden house overlooking the Bow River. The acres around had been left undeveloped; the river led to a creek that wound through ravines. I liked to walk there, studying the sky, which seemed lower than in my home town. Often birds circled above: hawks, crows, gulls. Always there was the dry scent of the prairie, grasses and sedges and brown earth. Once on a late fall afternoon I was standing at my favourite spot, high on a ravine overlooking the creek. Lost in reverie, I sensed something to my side and, shifting my eyes in that direction, looked to see what had caught my attention: a black wolf had come out of the scrub in the ravine to stand beside me. Its greyish nose, jet black nostrils atwitch, was no more than a foot from my knee. The wolf cut its eyes up to mine; it had sensed my look. We stood that way, studying each other for perhaps as long as a minute. Then the wolf twitched its tail and bounded away. I stood there for some time, experiencing an unusual wonder and inner peacefulness. A type of benediction had occurred. I had had no desire to touch the animal or communicate with it in any way; its mere presence, its otherness was what made the moment special. And yet there had been an acknowledgement in our mutual appraisal, a recognition of our separate but comparable existences, a sense of the beauty and majesty of life, whether lived by man or wolf. Whenever I have thought of that moment, the feeling of blessedness returns, a transcendent quietude akin to the *heart centre* of meditation. So I set out on a search for a spiritual healer. Calls to friends and then friends of friends yielded several names. But when I placed calls to these people, or tried to track them down in person—nothing. Phone calls were not returned; a mailed note seemed to have dropped into a black hole. (After repeated efforts I thought in a mood of some bemusement: perhaps they are not so much healers of the spirit as spirits that heal; they certainly did not appear to suffer the handicap of physical presence.)

For some years I had been visiting a massage therapist. EB had a treatment room in a building close to where I lived. His business card read: "Massage Therapy—Body, Mind, Spirit." He had been recommended by a friend during the period when my former wife and I were separating. EB is a stocky, muscular man of French Canadian descent. Once a business executive, he is admirably suited to the vocation he adopted later in life, after his own personal crisis. Even-tempered, responsive to the needs of others, quietly spiritual, professionally curious, and with powerful hands, EB creates an atmosphere of comfort and trust in his cozy treatment room. I had found his methods, especially his "cranial work," very liberating. In our early sessions he had helped me relax my muscles and release some deep-seated emotions as I opened myself to his low-key questions, his chatter, and his restorative touch. On several occasions I had left his treatment room feeling as well as I had felt as an adult: at peace and at the same time rejuvenated. I sometimes thought: EB helps me to see into myself, to relax with who I am, and to imagine who I could best be. He has made it possible for me to acknowledge my weaknesses and at the same time rebuild, using my strengths. In consequence, I had told EB that he was a fortunate man, able to help others through crises, a healer; to which he had modestly replied, "No, that's you; I'm just someone who helps along the way."

I recall that after I was diagnosed, I'd asked EB if he knew of a spiritual healer who might help me. "Hmm," he said, "not right off hand, but I'll think about it." Stocky though he is, EB seems to be a tall man, perhaps because he holds himself erect. He wears a trim beard, which he fingers when thinking. On that day I sensed some hesitation when I put my request to him. But he waved as he said goodbye on his doorstep, and repeated, "I'll give the spiritual healer thing some thought." Not long after I had occasion to visit him again. As he manipulated my shoulders he told me about a dying boy he'd been working with recently. The boy's condition had deteriorated rapidly; his parents had asked EB to come to the hospital in the last days to rub the child's neck and hold his hand in the final moments. He confided to me that he had sensed the second when the boy's soul had departed his body. EB paused after saying this and did not continue for a few minutes. Some days later, EB then reported, he had been strolling along the beach near his summer home, lost in

thought, when he felt a presence of unmistakable force sweep through him; his hair stood on end. He looked up and saw a white gull drifting by just above his head, and he thought, *that's H's soul.* And he'd been having that sensation ever since, sometimes experiencing an uncanny sense that H's soul was in the treatment room with him and whomever EB was attending to. As he talked, EB shook his head in wonder. I thought, *how open EB is to the emotional and spiritual vibrations of another's being.*

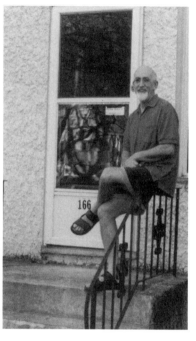

being. I had no wish to intrude on the moment. But I felt along with him the marvel of what he had experienced and the beauty of existence. I let EB rub the muscles on my shoulders and upper back. After a while I reached the point of inner peace, a sort of trance state akin to that achieved in meditation, when you are completely focussed and yet totally blank, your mind temporarily "free" and your body at ease in every respect. Then I had my own epiphany. I'd been searching for something I already had—a conduit to the spiritual world.

"EB," I said, "I've been stupidly blind about this, but it's clear to me now that you are my spiritual healer!" He chuckled, neither crediting the claim nor dismissing it. But I knew in that instant the truth of the realization. I felt it through my entire being, and was appalled that I had not realized it before. The problem was this: I had not been thinking of EB as a healer of the spirit. I had known for a long time that he was a healer, but in my simple-minded way I'd pigeonholed him— as massage therapist, and as a healer of the body only (I'd not seen the words "mind" and "spirit" on his card for years)—in the same manner I've spoken out against in this chapter when criticizing others. So. Shakespeare was right. There *is* more to life than is dreamt of in anyone's philosophy, mine included.

-By living through you I meant that I could live *with* cancer; I could, say, cook fine meals through cancer to proclaim the beauty of life and of living. Or I could write through cancer.

-You are going to die, dear boy.

-Everyone is going to die.

-You blather on. We are here, we exist; we will not go away.

-I concede that.

-So what's all this wind in the attic—what's the fuss?

-I could put the same question to you. Instead I'll say, it's like judo, or a martial art: use your opponent's strength against him. Undo him with his best weapon.

-Give over. You're muddying the waters with contradictions and paradoxes.

-You recommended the Buddha, remember?

-And am beginning to regret it.

-Use your adversary's force against him.

-Claptrap.

-Writing is an act of engaging cancer: as painting can be, or singing, or any one of dozens of other things. And not just the arts. Skiing, walking, jogging. You do these things not only for enjoyment. You write, for instance, to learn. You write to exorcise the demon.

-You cannot so easily rid yourself of us, you cannot spell us away.

-You look deep inside, you use words to bring the demon out into the open. Bringing the demon into the light diminishes it. You show it for what it is, and you weaken its grip on you. You deflate its power over you. It becomes just another *thing* that has befallen you—like losing your hair.

-We kill. We triumph. We are not rotten teeth.

-You are rotten luck. But you become silent in the face of the real facts: that you are just another bad thing to be lived through: like diabetes, or MS, or Crohn's. You are no greater than many other chronic diseases and life-long afflictions. You are *just* cancer.

-We concede nothing.

-You're becoming shrill.

-*We* prevail.

-Your strident claims resonate with alarm.

-Mutant cells *win.*

-We topple your hold over our imagination.

-Who is this *we?*

-We is those who experience the ride called Crazy Cancer Cruise. By bringing you out in the open through journals and diaries and written meditations we show your hold over us for what it is—Mister Oogey Boogey Man.

-Death?

-You've seen a windsock? When the wind suddenly shifts, it pops back through on itself, and what was outer becomes inner and vice versa. When we engage cancer rather than run from it, the same thing happens. We turn you inside out and see you for what you really are, and then you no longer frighten us.

-Crap.

-You lose your sting.

-Bull and nonsense.

-As you wish.

# Flickering Flame

*Lepidus Quintus Aemilius, going out of his house,*
*struck his big toe against the threshold and died.*

The meditation class was held at the University of Winnipeg, in a smallish lecture theatre designed for perhaps sixty. When I sat down near the back of the room, about half the spaces were taken. People seemed to have arrived in pairs and threes, little clusters whispering quietly. About five minutes after the appointed starting time a slim man in his mid-thirties with thinning blond hair walked to the front of the room. He was wearing blue jeans and a bulky Irish sweater. He was laughing and smiling as he placed the things he'd brought with him on the desk up front. He wrote his name on the board in chalk: G.

G told us he was there to teach us about meditation. We were to learn about it as he had from the master named Sri Chimoy. He wrote this name on the board, too. G told us that *yoga* was an all-purpose word for every kind of meditation, not just for the type he referred to as physical meditation, yoga exercises. He told us there were a number of steps to learning meditation. He wrote the word *concentration* on the board and talked about it. It was the first of seven steps in meditation, G explained. Some of the others were *relaxation* and *mantra*. He said Sri Chimoy had told him, "I meditate to free my mind." Words flowed out of G easily. Sometimes he talked about himself: he'd abandoned a career in real estate; he wanted to be a writer. At other times he talked about the difficulties of meditation; and at others about his master, Sri Chimoy, who, G claimed, could lift enormous weight because he harnessed such great concentration. G said we were aiming for a version of that concentration called "heart centre."

He looked about the room from time to time—institutional grey walls, plastic desks arranged in rows, tile on the floor, fluorescent tubing overhead. Not the most inviting environment for journeys into the depths of one's inner self.

G had come into the room carrying a number of books and a small bag, like the airlines used to give away to fliers. He sat on the edge of the desk on the raised dais at the front of the room. He laughed about showing up late for our session that morning. "There's two kinds of time," he explained, "ordinary time and meditation time." He told us that he always had to explain to his friends which kind of time he was operating under on any given occasion. From the bag G produced a candle and a small candle holder. These he placed on the desk. He had talked up to that point about many things, including the mind, which he called "the beast," because it was always gobbling up things like time and wanting to have everything for itself. G fiddled with the candle until it stood up on its own in the candle holder. He had spent a lot of time talking about concentration, but now, he said, it was time to actually do some concentrating. He lit the candle, and then he shut off the lights in the lecture theatre. Focus on the candle, he told us, and think only of the dancing flame. We tried. It seemed easy. After about half a minute G said, "That's easy, see. The trick is to be able to do that for extended periods of time."

We tried concentrating on the candle for a minute or so. He was right. The mind jumped around. One moment you were thinking about the flickering flame and the next you

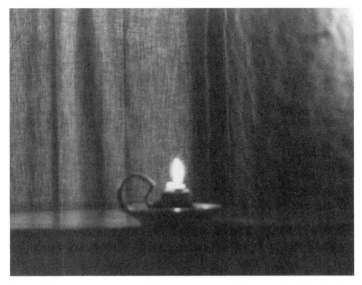

found that you were recalling a conversation you had had that morning without ever being aware that your thinking had jumped from the one to the other. It was difficult to keep such a fine focus that you never lost the flame. G laughed and said we had to learn to free the mind from itself. He went on to explain to us what he called "the flick." Whenever we sensed that our mind was about to drift off the candle and onto something else, we were to flick away whatever had popped into our mind. He mimicked one of us thinking to ourselves, "Now what was it they said about the weather for tomorrow on the radio?"—and then he snapped his fingers and said, "flick." We practised that, too. Concentrate. Sense the mind, the beast, about to leap. Flick. After twenty minutes or so it was becoming easier to maintain concentration for a minute and more. But it was also not easy to focus so intensely for long periods of time. G explained that we were not to be vexed about that. "Total focus," he explained, "really meditating, comes and goes in waves." He made a motion in the air with his hand, a rollercoaster. We had to learn to ride out the moments when we lost focus and ready ourselves for the next. We had to learn patience and humour about what we were doing. "Maybe," G said, "this candle does not work for some of you, and if so, you close your eyes and try thinking of a candle flame in the mind."

So it went. We practised meditating for short periods, and in between these brief periods of experiment with yoga, G talked about what meditation had done for some people—himself included—and about meditation as a way of life. People the world over had turned to meditation in times of anxiety and disaster and trauma, and they'd found an inner strength in meditating that helped them cope with these personal crises. They were, in his words, "more together" people. They had experienced a shift in values (for some a minor shift, for others, quite major). Many no longer put so much emphasis on being the top dog or on climbing the ladder of success or on having possessions, and so on. Others had healed inner wounds and were able to reconnect with family members after years of separation. So meditation could be a very potent agency for goodness. But also, G cautioned, meditation is not a panacea for whatever has gone awry in our lives; it is, though, a very effective way of coming to fundamental understandings about ourselves that might help in re-focussing our lives.

About two hours into the session we attempted a longer meditation. Like the mental *beast* of most of the others present in the room, I assumed, my mind wandered from the candle after a minute or so, but it came back to the candle, too, and about fifteen minutes into the session I felt my eyes (pinched somewhat together in what G called "the lion's stare") begin to water slightly and my breathing to come in deep tranquil rhythms. Quite unexpectedly, something in my chest gave way and for a minute or so I felt a wonderful quietude and peace come over me; in that brief period I no longer had to focus on the candle flame, but was, in fact, completely focussed on it and nothing else. Effortlessly. Focussed without trying, it seemed. It was a trance-like twinkling of time, no more than a minute or so, and it passed. But I knew when G flicked on the light in the room that I had experienced "heart centre," that I had meditated. I felt freed and totally engaged, at once.

For about a year and a half after being diagnosed I meditated daily. I became quite accomplished at achieving heart centre, a deep peace that begins in the chest cavity and that spreads throughout the body, manifesting itself most obviously as slackening in the eye muscles and tranquil and rhythmic breathing. When we travelled to other cities and to Europe, I carried a candle and matches with me. Meditation was a special and important time in every day for me. I sensed that it was all about breathing, about learning to hear every fibre of your body vibrate with the goodness of *OHM* and *AUM*.

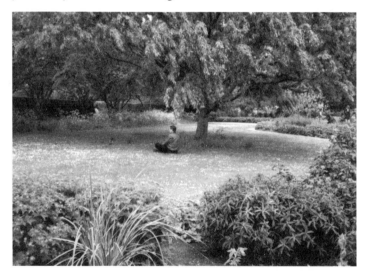

G had told us that meditation was particularly effective in easing stress. I had always had a low heart rate, but he was right about that in other ways than the one merely associated with slowing down. Meditation taught me to be peaceful within myself and with my self. Without teaching me anything specific about life—how to be gentler with those around me, for instance—it had (and continues to have) that effect on my behaviour. It is a *spot* in most of my days, an oasis of a sort where I slow down and turn inward and come to peace with myself and my condition. From out of that "spot" flows a mood that sustains me for hours, a mood in which the things that ordinarily provoke me and cause me anxiety wash off me in a bubbling cascade. Conversely, it creates in me a positive mood, one in which I am more likely to perform small, unremembered acts of kindness and of love. So yoga is not only a haven, a step back from the workaday world, a retreat, but something that makes it possible for me to return to my everyday life renewed and refreshed and able to be a stronger and yet gentler person. Not easy things to achieve—and not easy things to write about without sensing that you're drifting into a certain kind of casuistry. But it works. I am grateful to G for teaching me. Like a number of people I have encountered since being diagnosed, G is out there helping others in his serene, self-effacing, bulky Irish sweater way, a considerate man and a helpful one, who has as his reward for his kindness to others not wealth and fame, but his own heart centre.

Meditation is probably not for everyone. Nor is visualization, a technique of total focus that sets as its goal everything from the easing of anxiety in moments of stress to actual interference in one's physical state. You've probably seen athletes at a big meet standing in front of the high bar or the run-up to the pit and mentally rehearsing each step they are about to take. This strategy of mental focus can produce remarkable results, both on the field of competition and off. Bernie Siegel says in one of his books that he has known patients who practised visualization to limit the amount of bleeding they did when under anaesthetic in surgery. Many patients have attested to the power of the mind in working to right a physical wrong (such as tension in the shoulders or back pain). Carl Simonton claims that patients who visualize the healthy cells in their bodies attacking the cancerous ones live longer and fuller lives than those who do not. No less of an authority in this area than Norman Cousins claims that recovery arises from one's inner disposition to disease and the healing process: every patient, he contends, carries his own doctor inside. There are many—and among them large numbers who do not suffer from a serious disease—who swear by visualization and practise it every day of their lives. It takes some time to learn, and it's not easy to find the time every day to do, but it can be truly effective in dealing with one's condition. At the very least visualization is worth a try. My older sister uses it to reduce stress when she comes home from work; when K senses a sore throat coming on—prelude to a flu attack in these parts—she takes several caps of vitamin C, visualizes the antioxidants attacking the germ cells, and, in a high percentage of cases, avoids that bout of influenza.

In my own case, visualization came to comprise the following routine: sitting comfortably in my meditation position, I rivet my attention on relaxing the muscles in my body, systematically working from those of the scalp, through the temple, the jaw, and so on, down to the intestines and even farther. When I feel completely at one with myself, I begin to visualize the killer-T cells in my arteries, imagining them moving through the bloodstream, seeking out, and then pouncing on the cancer cells in the tumours in my liver (I saw a film clip about this, quite graphic, and I rehearse what I'd viewed in the clip—fierce killer-T cells attacking and destroying aberrant cells). With my eyes closed and mentally intent on the visual combat I conjure up, I recapitulate this scenario for some ten or fifteen minutes at a stretch, sensing as I do so how these intense psychic acts support the functioning of the physiological process taking place in my body. I feel good about the experience, feel I am complementing the work of the interferon in my system, feel I'm taking an important step toward health. Visualization is a strategy I can put to work for myself.

But. For a brief period of months I had to give up visualization and meditation. Being a committed believer in the power of the mind, I made it a regular daily routine to meditate for a half hour and then to practise visualization in the half hour immediately following that. This worked in the short term, bringing a number of positive results and feelings. Perhaps the early success was a bit of a curse. The success encouraged me to really work at visualization. I discovered in the long run, though, that so much intense concentration was having a negative effect, too. Internally I was "tying myself up," and one result was a physiological one: my intestines sometimes felt tense and knotted, I became mildly nauseous. Then constipated. So I backed off the practice of meditating followed by visualization. I gave myself a time out from intense mental activity. Cancer, it can be said with no exaggeration, is a consuming disease; it feels as if it's consuming our bodies. But equally it can be a consuming ailment in a mental way, occupying our minds and thoughts so fully that it ends up endangering our psyches, too.

So sitting quietly and "thinking" your way through an ailment may not be the route for everyone, but it can be effective. The same can be said of prayer. Raised a Lutheran, I went through the motions of praying for much of my early life: the Lord's Prayer, the Creeds of the Apostles, and so on. Mouthed the words until I was fifteen or so and then drifted away from Church and God and prayer. Not an unusual scenario. Prayer is a kind of conversation with God—with something greater than us, anyway. I have learned to see prayer that way since contracting cancer. I have prayed in desperation—as we all must do in moments of deep fright (you remember the quip, "There are no atheists in foxholes"). But I have also learned to "pray" for guidance from that larger-thing-than-us (God), to ask for greater insight into my condition and my life and my sometimes erratic and hurtful behaviour. Just humbling oneself this way, just forming the words opens the door, I have learned, to first understanding and then improvement. We're so reluctant to relinquish pride. Like meditation, prayer is a way of moving deep inside the self to see the self at its nakedest, weakest, and most frightened, and—paradoxically—to stand momentarily outside the self and imagine how things could be different. You do not have to be in any real sense religious to pray, and you may not become religious if you do pray—if by religion you mean the trappings of churches and creeds and the like—but if you pray you will become more spiritual. That's nothing to fear.

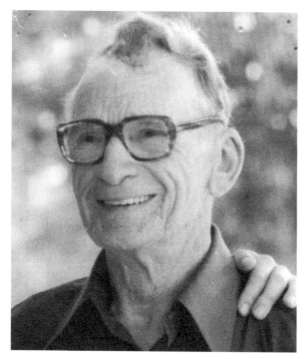

After he died, my father's tools came into my possession. Sometimes I find myself in the basement, handling a hammer or a power drill or a screwdriver, and I hear myself saying, "Oh, Dad." The mental picture of my father the last time I saw him alive, wearing a brown and green cardigan sweater, waving from the doorway as I drove away, comes back to me. I hear myself saying half aloud, "We miss you, Dad," or "I'm trying to be as good a father to my son as you were to yours." These utterances, addressed partly to ourselves, partly to loved ones no longer with us, are prayers of a kind: acknowledgments of our debt to those who have gone before us, and requests for guidance from their presences, and optimistic asides that we hope will improve our outlook on life and affect our behaviour. Prayers to "God" are similar: utterances that proceed from various needs and that feel as much like reminders to ourselves to be strong and courageous as they feel like appeals to a higher being to do things *for* us.

Going down into yourself in the way of meditation, visualization, and prayer was not easy for me. Each requires that paradoxical combination of intense concentration and mental letting go that leads to epiphanies and insights. At first focussing this way proved frustrating; progress was slow. Like most things that are worth doing, spiritual exercises require a lot of practice and patience. Also I may have resisted the spiritual side of these practices for another reason. Meditation, visualization, and prayer each, in its own way, requires a humbling of the self before the complexities and mysteries of the cosmos. For these techniques to succeed, I had to learn to confess—even if only to myself—weakness and vulnerability. Furthermore, I had to accept that to improve my situation required examining my whole life, and there was a part of me that preferred not to take that unsettling step. At a number of points I had to admit I'd made mistakes—like hurting loved ones—in the past, and to acknowledge that it was time to make amends. Such undertakings require relinquishing control of our everyday selves and submitting the self to close scrutiny. For me, as for many others, such acknowledgements were disturbing, and they required quite a bit of emotional effort.

The reward of such humbling of the self is the opening up of the lines of communication within yourself. You know how it is when someone is talking just to hear themselves talk—blah blah blah—but not saying anything? That's a monologue that just happens to have the luxury of a listener, not a dialogue. A dialogue has two sides and fosters a mutual exchange. If you're like me, you probably have talks with yourself, arguing through both sides of an issue or a dispute. We learn from such exchanges, by playing out both sides, airing a number of positions. In such inner dialogues we discover things we did not know we knew, or at least the terms that express them most fittingly and usefully. Often we arrive at resolutions this way, sometimes closure. But even this kind of conversation, or talking to yourself, works best when you actually listen to yourself and take up the issues that are generated by the other voices in inner dialogue—rather than just venting your favourite prejudices. You have to hear your self, your better self, just as you have to hear others in a conversation. Odd as it may at first sound, in order to live through cancer, you have to learn to have a relationship with yourself.

Improvements in our physical condition develop slowly. Rarely do we undergo a procedure that miraculously alters our health for the better. That usually comes in slow increments, which build on one another, sometimes as a result of a process that feels as if every two steps forward come at the cost of one step back. Earlier in these pages I mentioned the biblical story of Saul on the road to Damascus. It's an inspiring story, the tale of sudden and amazing conversion, but it's not true to the life most of us lead. Our lives build on incremental repetitions that lead to improvement over time. Healing, emotional and spiritual, works the same way. We gather strength in small ways; we acquire insights that build one on another, rarely in a blinding flash of light. The healing journey resembles the prolonged and sometimes exasperating trek of Moses through the deserts more than that of Saul on the road to Damascus.

Healing comes to us in all kinds of ways. The drugs we take combat the diseases we have contracted; the treatments we undergo shift the toxic imbalances in our bodies; surgery can eliminate a lesion that is metastasizing and producing others; herbal remedies introduce doses of products into our bodies that readjust our organic chemistry; massage therapy eases our muscles and gives us a more relaxed attitude to everyday life; psychic therapy helps us deal with the issues raised by our ailments. And so on down the line. Healing is not one-dimensional. The resources are all around us—concoctions created to address physiological needs, acupuncture, group chanting, and many more. Meditation, visualization, and prayer are three avenues to the power of the mind, that silent partner of the body that can be turned to positive achievements. You've no doubt encountered the concept that human beings use only a small portion of their brains. Meditation, visualization, and prayer tap some of the other portions of our mental capacities, guiding us to the inner self and helping us to heal that self as well as to heal its partner organic element that we call our bodies. Some physicians and most practitioners of alternative medicine claim that no healing can occur without the right mental disposition in the patient. Though we cannot heal ourselves, we can create better conditions for healing to occur; through mental acts we can open ourselves to the range of healing possibilities and then let those possibilities flourish as they will.

-You're a gas bag, dear boy, a pompous one at that.

-Name-calling, I will not bite on that.

-Your ego is something else, you know? You understand one thing, one small thing, and your head swells up like a balloon.

-I will not be taken in by your name-calling and shabby jibes; I will not be provoked because—

-Then listen to the facts. You have cancer. That is your reality.

-That is one of my realities. Another is that I have caring friends. Another that I have a loving wife; another a joyous son; another a happy family. Shall I go on?

-Give us a break.

-It's a long list. It includes prayer and meditation and cycling and walks and laughing at Bill Cosby and massage therapy and reading a good book.

-Cancer.

-It includes cross-country skiing and singing along to Stan Rogers and taking all day to make timballo del gatopardo for friends.

-We get the last word: Death.

-That famous last word is no more than a pathetic sop: because in the end, it's not about winning.

-"Succumbed to cancer," your obituary will read.

-"Loved his family; played tennis; cycled in Europe."

-Oh, do give over. You're like a teenager who has discovered the pleasures of the body: you can't stop playing with yourself; you can't stop going on about it.

-"Published a dozen books; built a wine cellar."

-You bore us to tears. Go away.

-As you will.

# Treadmills

*You must change your life.*

—Rainer Maria Rilke

Being diagnosed with cancer can feel like taking a hard punch to the solar plexus: for a period of time—weeks, even months—you stagger around with the wind knocked out of you, emotionally speaking. You feel lost; you feel unfocussed; defeated. The dread of dying falls over you like a dark shadow and when it lifts, it is replaced by a profound inertia. You cannot help thinking, *What's the point?* Everything that you were planning has come to ashes; the future you anticipated unravels before your eyes. The life you were leading seems suddenly to be pointless and the value of going on evaporates.

In the western world we are, for a large part of our lives, motivated by goals—often *driven* is more accurate. We strive to succeed at our work, to accumulate wealth, to raise a happy family, to be somebody. We look forward to being in a position of power, or to earning flattering remuneration, or to seeing our children succeed, or to retirement. We scud along at our occupations and in our families, more or less happy with our lot in life and content with who we are, building a life.

Without quite knowing it, we embrace the poet's dictum that "a man's reach should exceed his grasp." Then we learn that we have a life-threatening illness, and the wind is knocked out of our sails.

In short, having led a life of achievement can be a kind of curse. Being motivated toward high goals has many obvious benefits: achievement, success, self-worth, wealth. But it also has a down side. When those high goals seem inaccessible, it's possible to plunge into a serious downdraft. High goals can cast a dark cloud over our sense of self-worth when—or if— we no longer sense we can achieve them.

It's easy in the period immediately following diagnosis to give up—on oneself, on one's family, on one's work. Physical debilitation and mental exhaustion combine to sap our energy. Treatments, especially chemotherapy, wear the body down; nothing seems more welcome than prolonged retirement from the workaday world and profound rest. Our physiognomy changes—sometimes dramatically. We lose hair, our skin turns grey, pounds drop off our bones. We are not happy with what we see in the mirror, and we tremble to go out into the world to be seen by those who knew us when we were robust and healthy. In addition, many of us think we have become mere shadows of our former selves. Where before we could consume large meals, work long hours, and engage in strenuous physical activity, we now find ourselves easily tired and frighteningly short of the energy that powered our lives only a short time before. We may think, *I'm only half the person I used to be.* We may be tempted to give up because we are no longer the vigorous specimen we once were. And thoughts of that kind spin us downward into despondency, depression, and despair.

This is a crucial period in one's experience with cancer. At this time we must make a concerted effort to grit our teeth and re-engage life. This is where goals serve a critical purpose. Goals, even when we have a terminal illness, give us something to look forward to, give us the strength to go on minute by minute, day by day, and year by year. They turn our thinking outward, away from our debilitating condition and on to life-enhancing aspects of experience such as family, outings, accomplishments, and friends. In short, goals make the future possible by being the future we can envision and pursue. And without some notion of future we ordinary human beings have a very difficult time going on from day to day.

But—there's always a *but*, isn't there?—it may be important, possibly critical, in the period directly following diagnosis to redefine one's goals. To transform them.

It can be difficult immediately after being diagnosed to maintain goals, or to even imagine having goals. I recall thinking almost instantly after I was told *you have cancer* that my son, then aged three, would grow up without a father. Raising our children is a goal we pretty much take for granted. But I was devastated by this thought. I pictured my boy going through his formative years without me, and the images I conjured cut deeply. It was weeks before I understood my condition better and set an ambitious but tantalizing goal for myself: to see him graduate from high school. To that one simple but enticing objective I have since added a number of other goals: to re-establish contact with neglected friends, to visit certain places, to complete the writing of specific books, and so on.

These are ambitious goals, long-term objectives that I hope to achieve. At first it is wiser to set somewhat more limited goals. This can be difficult, especially for those of us who are used to working hard and achieving a lot. In the first flush to beat cancer, our initial response to rehabilitation may be to set our goals too high; we may think that if we strenuously resist cancer, we can deliver it a knockout blow and defeat it wholly and quickly. And that can be a terrible error in judgement, leading to the exhaustion of our resources and further debilitation of our bodies. The more sensible thing is to set goals well within our reach. (That way we can gauge what the outside limits of our strength are and we can learn to work within these: much better that than to exhaust our bodies, or to be frustrated by objectives that are no longer within our grasp.)

Carl Simonton suggests making a grid or graph for oneself: on it he recommends placing daily goals (such as eating one good meal), and weekly goals (walking a specific distance outdoors, say), and monthly goals, and so on. Setting these simple goals serves a number of functions: they keep us focussed on things we *can* accomplish, rather than on what we can no longer do. They give us a purpose; they give us a future. If you construct such a grid for yourself, you may find that ticking off the items you accomplish—whether on paper or only in the mind—serves an important psychological function. Checking these goals off when we've achieved them sustains us in a significant way: it cultivates a sense of accomplishment, an important psychological boost in a forbidding period of one's life when it probably seems that nothing can anymore be accomplished. This is as true of very minor goals as well as the major ones: even sitting up in bed, or reading a chapter of a book, or talking on the phone can be a satisfying achievement at certain points in one's cancer journey.

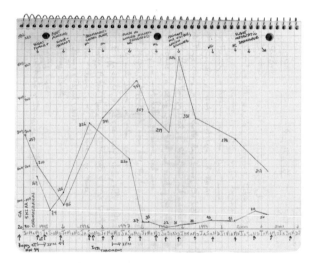

Whatever goals you set for yourself, and however you go about achieving them, the most significant thing here is balance. Nearly everyone agrees that living with cancer (and surviving cancer) requires a certain amount of dedication to the task of surviving cancer. It requires a forward-looking attitude, commitment to objectives, a sense of the future. It's important to have goals, then, but not to have goals come to dominate one's daily experience. In our society we like to keep records of things. The sports world these days seems dominated by statistics: salaries, goals, wins, and so on. Those of us not in the sports world have our own versions of these statistics: years on the job, salary, days without missing work. These objective measurements build up our sense of self-worth and document the fact that we have done things, ultimately that we are here, that we *are*. In that climate it can be easy to slip into certain errors of proportion: we can make goals so important that they become more significant than just living, just enjoying experiences that present themselves in and for themselves. Furthermore, people diagnosed with cancer may fall into the trap of setting goals and then equating the achieving of those goals with beating cancer (that equation may occur in the unconscious, not the conscious mind); but whatever the case, achieving those goals is not necessarily beating cancer: all one has done is achieve the goals.

I encountered a cancer patient some years ago who told me this cautionary tale. CB was a former athlete. Shortly after diagnosis she set herself the goal of working out for twenty minutes every day. She had been accustomed to an hour and a half. In her mind, CB confessed, an unconscious equation took shape: doing the workout came to mean winning the battle against cancer. So she developed a routine: pounding on the treadmill, pumping iron, pedaling a bicycle, climbing the Stairmaster. She sweated; she trained; she stuck to the program. Then one day in the middle of her routine, she collapsed and found herself later in the infirmary with cold compresses on her forehead. She had prostrated herself with exertion. In the determination to beat cancer, CB had exhausted herself, punishing her body in the effort to render it more healthy. Ironically, she'd enslaved herself to a short-term goal that was defeating her larger overall purpose—quality health and quality living.

In the chapter entitled "Meditation, Visualization, and Prayer," I briefly document how meditating and visualizing for an hour every day (a goal I set for myself early in my healing journey) actually "back-fired" on me, causing me physical discomfort instead of helping achieve the goals of relaxation and defeating cancer, which were the goals I had set for myself. This is an easy trap to fall into. We are eager to prove that we are beating the disease, that we are winning. Another chapter identifies one thing as being the most important in the cancer journey: re-inventing oneself. That means seeing oneself anew and reassessing one's experience: recognizing the bounds of our energy and acknowledging the limits that a life-threatening disease has set on our human duration; but also recognizing where there are possibilities of growth, of being more than you were before cancer.

Raised in the fifties, I had been taught that my duties as a man were to be a good breadwinner and strong family head. For that you needed to be successful. Like most men of my generation, I worked long hours and over time achieved the success that was expected of us: house in the suburbs, cars, bank account, and so on. Though not blindly ambitious, nor ruthless in my climb up the organizational ladder, I had followed a typical course for men of my generation. At the workplace my counsel was sought, my advice heeded; I was offered promotions, and I accumulated wealth. I was proud of these things; they showed I had made something of myself. I associated these things with masculinity and became a model of "masculine" success. But I had neglected other things in my life: I was closed off emotionally; I rarely exposed vulnerability, and I regarded evidence of it in others as signs of personal weakness, as an indication of failure. In terms of sympathy, compassion, and openness, I remained undeveloped—or underdeveloped.

In specific terms, re-inventing myself has meant—and continues to mean—seeing myself as different from before diagnosis. I can no longer afford the luxury of being the "strong silent man," Gary Cooper in the suburbs. I have had

to acknowledge weakness and vulnerability in my body and in my character. I'm a man with cancer, a cancer that will kill me. In many ways, I no longer want to be The Man. A part of me winces to write this sentence, but here's a list of the ways in which I have changed—and am trying to change—as I re-invent myself after diagnosis:
- eat better, drink less, take herbal supplements;
- not push myself too hard physically;
- acknowledge earlier ambitions and reassess them;
- look inside myself to try to understand my self;
- place more value on loving and on loved ones;
- take time to revel in life's sensual aspects;
- acknowledge how I regarded others' needs as weaknesses;
- recognize vulnerability and weakness in myself;
- talk over issues rather than close off communication;
- express emotions more freely and more openly;
- recognize the place of the spiritual in daily life;
- embrace grace from others when encountered;
- accept that I may have to make amends for earlier hurtful behaviour;
- humble myself before others.

As I say, these are not reflections that I comfortably commit to publication; and these have not been easy acknowledgements for a man raised in my time and place to affirm. Yet they are my new goals because they are intimately tied up with re-inventing my self and with healing. In brief, I know now that to the extent that we are able to transform the earlier objectives we set ourselves, as well as transforming our notions of who we are and how we live, to that extent will our living through cancer be a positive experience.

-Listen. Once upon a time—

-Oh, really.

-Once upon a time, I took things for granted—a good meal, the love of friends, joyful sex, a fall sunset; all that wonderful stuff that goes into a full but unrealized life. Yes?

-You're full of yourself, dear boy.

-You came into my life—into my guts—and I had to change.

-You could no longer go on being the clown you were.

-Change. And not just in the obvious sense, the physical sense.

-Hair loss, grey skin, flushing, diarrhea: what is all that? That mattered to you?

-Quite a lot. But here's the point. I had to re-assess myself and then re-invent myself.

-Give over with the psycho-babble.

-You forced me to become someone I was not before. In obvious ways, yes. By slowing down, by not taking that sunset for granted. That way. Also by learning to be more kind, more gentle, more reflective.

-Oh, this is too much. Touchy-feely, you know?

-There's more. I've had to look back on my past and recognize that I was often a jerk—that I hurt people. I have had to acknowledge that and then seek forgiveness for it. Humble myself. My Self. To humble myself; to submit myself to trust when I did not even comprehend what I was trusting in.

-You do rattle the windowpanes with your fifty-buck words.

-I had to grasp the fact that I was indeed going to die—probably of cancer—and that it was up to me to make my dying (as well as the living I had left) mean something. To be someone who could die, rather than have Death come upon them.

-You do blather on, dear boy.

# Dropped Fork, Slurped Soup

*Getting cancer was the best thing that happened to me.*

—Lance Armstrong

It's a late Friday afternoon in November and I'm lying on the floor in our living room, curled up into a foetal ball. My son is in the family room, playing video games. K is puttering about the house, watering plants. It's my birthday and I'm fifty-three. What an irony! This should be an "up" day. BUT. There used to be a little boy who came to summer camp with the other tykes in the old *Peanuts* comic strip; he went immediately to his bunk, turned his back on whomever was in the room with him and stated, "Leave me alone." This is precisely how I feel. *Noli me tangere.* I'm down.

Nothing in particular has happened to plummet me into this state of funk. About two weeks earlier I had gone in for a regularly scheduled CT scan of my bowel. A week later I met with Doctor AM, who informed me the tumours in my liver were stable. He was pleased by the radiologist's report. So was I. Good news for a cancer patient is the news that the disease has not progressed. Though there had been a few

133

uncomfortable moments in the clinic on the day of the CT scan, they were no longer bothering me. For a week I had been feeling good about things in general. On a couple of nights I had not slept well, true—rumbling guts. I had taken the mild tranquilizer lorazepam one night and felt a little muzzy the following morning. But that was fairly typical.

So what was the problem?

Cancer tumours throw all kinds of chemicals into our bloodstream. Mostly the deleterious by-products of cancer are hormones—among them serotonin. (Other products are peptides and tachykinins.) These chemicals pollute our bodies and sometimes have the effect of over-loading our systems

April 03, 2000

## A "Direct Hit" Against Liver Tumors

HealthNews from the publishers of *The New England Journal of Medicine*

In more than half of the nearly 130,000 Americans diagnosed with colorectal cancer each year, the disease eventually spreads (metastasizes) to the liver. Treatment at that point typically involves surgery to remove liver tumors, but liver metastases usually recur within two years.

A new strategy to reduce recurrence and improve survival for people with liver tumors arising from colorectal cancer turns the cancer's method of nourishment against itself. Noting that liver tumors draw their blood supply primarily from the hepatic artery while normal liver cells get theirs from a different blood vessel, researchers at Memorial Sloan-Kettering Cancer Center in New York devised a way to feed cancer-fighting drugs directly to the tumor through the hepatic artery.

In a study reported in the Dec. 30, 1999 *New England Journal of Medicine*, 74 patients with colorectal cancer that had spread to the liver had a small pump surgically implanted to provide chemotherapy directly to the hepatic artery. All these patients also had traditional systemic chemotherapy. Meanwhile, 82 similar patients had standard chemotherapy alone.

Among patients with the pump (called hepatic arterial infusion therapy), the survival rate after two years was 86 percent, compared with 72 with elements that have a powerful negative effect on our health. We become internally awash in a kind of poisonous bath—and without even knowing that it's happening! Add to this the depressive effects of tranquilizers and you're looking at a formula for despondency—if not worse. One morning, one afternoon, some evening, we're abruptly subject to a dark mood, which, as time passes, becomes darker and darker. These violent plummets into black funks, these "attacks," are sudden, random, and unpredictable. We become testy; we become short-tempered with our loved ones; we hate them and we hate the world at large; and we also hate ourselves. We're in the throes of depression.

I used to think that people who were depressed were depressed *about* something—a traumatic event, bad news, a failure at work, a slight from someone, unremitting pain. To remedy depression, I thought, you would merely change these exterior circumstances—see the grave news in a better light, for instance—and the depression would lift. Depression does not work that way. Depression is something that comes at you without your even knowing about it. You think maybe that it began with a physical effect, but then it seems not so much physical as psychological. Outside or inside? It's impossible to tell. What you do know is that a terrible thing has settled over you—and you cannot shake it loose. Depression infiltrates you. It inhabits your being rather than merely afflicting you, in the same way a virus inhabits your body. Depression announces itself as a dark cloud that is suddenly inside your skull, blackening everything you perceive; and it's such an intense presence that it is difficult sometimes to grasp that others cannot see it. It replaces who you have been and becomes who you *are*. Depression is a stain that spreads out into your entire being. It takes over. It is the only reality you know. It seems it has a life of its own. You can grow so used to its presence that you may be surprised when someone near to you cannot sense it the way you do, as an actual thing, hovering near. Others may try to shake you loose from it but that is nearly always futile. You cannot be joked out of it. You cannot be diverted by the tricks used to divert upset children. You might as well try to stop the snow from falling outside as stop another person's depression. You might as well try to reverse the flood waters in a gorge by holding up your hands.

Has anyone ever been able to stop someone who is intent on suicide?

Depression is a demon. When you're lying on the floor curled up in a foetal ball everything seems pointless. If your spouse dares to ask, "Can I get you anything?" you answer in an impatient, barely audible, and surly voice, "No." In fact, during a state of depression, a down period, monosyllables are the order of communication. About the most you can manage is, "Go away. Leave me alone." You've probably seen a cat or a dog when it becomes very sick. Only yesterday filled with energy and perky to the call, they grow completely listless; they find a corner in the room or in the garage or under the verandah; they curl up into a ball and lie silently, eyes glazed over, breathing through the mouth, tongue protruding. I don't know if dogs experience depression—probably not— but these are the classic symptoms that manifest themselves in humans. In me anyway.

*Noli me tangere.* Don't touch me.

Suicidal thoughts.

Unforgivable behaviour.

During more than one of these episodes I have lashed out at K, hurting her beyond the point where she was willing to say to A, "It's just the cancer talking," their typical way of excusing my dark moods. As I lay on the couch festering and spoiling, thoughts came to me from my conversations with FS, the psychiatrist, especially his concern about K. I grasped then what I had not understood earlier. He had anticipated these moments of suppressed rage, of depression; and he had thought perhaps they were already on us, and was concerned about how K would weather them. She was holding up and so was I—but the black moods brought with them ugly behaviour and a terrible inner struggle.

This may sound self-pitying and self-indulgent. You may

be tempted to think, *all you need to do is get a grip on yourself and get on with life.* Someone less charitable might think, *what this person needs is a good boot in the butt.* There was a time when I might have held that opinion myself.

On certain occasions there is an objective reality to one's state of melancholy. At the clinic you are sometimes told that the tumours have grown. You feel defeated: all the injections with interferon, all the thoughtful eating, all the exercise, the positive thoughts, the meditation, the prayers, the vitamin C, and yet the tumours have grown. You cannot believe your ears; you leave the clinic in a funk. Depression hovers. Or the oncologist

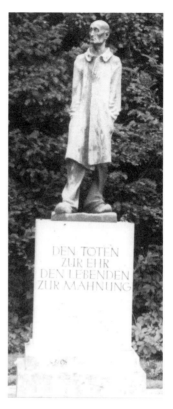

notices that your liver is not precisely where it is on healthy people, that yours is several centimetres below your rib cage. The observation provokes a certain amount of prodding and poking. Other physicians are brought into the consulting room, stethoscopes appear. You ask, *does this indicate that my liver is failing?* "Just a moment," the physician says and disappears to consult. Yet when he returns, he does not answer your question, but instead examines your back and listens to your heart. "Your liver has fallen," you are told—and as an afterthought, "fallen slightly." What does that mean? You leave the clinic still wondering: "Is my liver failing?" Despondent. Or you find yourself flushing more than usual. Not just when you have an alcoholic drink, but frequently. You rise in the morning and check yourself in the mirror: what was once an irregular flushing that covered your entire face and then sub-sided—like a blush—has become a permanent discolouration about the size of a hockey puck. Or there are pains, there are aches, there is surgery, followed by more pain. There are days of painkillers and physical immobility and strained and enforced patience. These things throw you into a deep funk. Your blood work comes back with higher (or lower) levels than on previous occasions. Things are going amiss inside you; chemicals are brewing; your immune system is having to battle alarming battalions of radical cells. You try not to find yourself staring out the window, seemingly blank. How many more times will you see the lilacs come into bloom; how many more Boxing Days will be spent cross-country skiing in the park with your wife and son?

When you visit a doctor of sport medicine with a twisted ankle, he sends you for X-ray and then tests, in case there's some connection to your cancer. If you tumble off your mountain bike when negotiating an off-road route and injure your lower back, you are sent for a bone scan—in case there has been metastasis. This enrages you. You are not a bloody invalid! And yet you are perceived as fragile—and you are.

You are sick. You have cancer. You are dying.

Down is a vortex, a vortex that I can feel myself spinning downwards in, but am powerless to arrest. Down is a vortex with no bottom. Soon small things will prove irritable in the extreme—a dropped fork at the dinner table, say. Soon I will blame others for minor gaffes that occur around the house: a flapping screen door, or someone slurping their soup. I will rage over trivialities but not in the way that leads to venting and healing. I will hold the anger in, and soon there will be seething, and then I will become even more withdrawn: surly, unresponsive, and finally plain miserable. I know that in addition to being uncommunicative, surly, and brusque, these will seem minor darknesses compared to others that will move in like storm clouds. I will become mean. I will say I no longer see the point of life. I will tell K: "If I knew how to tell A goodbye, I would bring it to an end."

I will lash out at those I love. I will make them feel the pain I feel.

Cancer consumes: it eats up our bodies and takes over our psyches.

In the throes of depression I want to scream, I want to throw things, I want to bash my hockey stick on the ground until my arms grow weak from fatigue. I do these things. They do not help.

Depression is a sickness. It sucks all the beauty out of the world, all the hope, and what remains is death-in-life, a joyless and suffocating nullity. After a few days of it I also feel physically terrible—headache, gut pains, listlessness. But unlike other ailments, which cause measurable pain that has a finite duration, depression leads me to believe that I'm just tired—or strung out, or having a bad mood. In brief, down.

I know all this, but knowing it doesn't change anything. None of it explains what depression is. Or more important, how to rise above it.

You may remember a book popular in the sixties, Richard Farina's *Been Down So Long It Looks Like Up to Me.* Farina documents accurately how we spin out of our usual temperament in depressive moments and how difficult it is to right ourselves. He had no lasting solution to the problem, and I have no magic remedy, either. Recognizing that you are in a state of depression helps. It helps to keep you from displacing your anger on to others—and lashing out at them. You may realize that what is actually bothering you is not the dropped fork, or the banging door, or the sound of slurped soup. Perhaps it is only the deadly mixture of chemicals coursing through your system. But recognizing that will not change the mood. It may only spare someone dear to you the brunt of your wrath. There are strategies you may try: going out for a long walk may ameliorate the situation—may. On occasion you can walk yourself out of a black hole: physical exertion can burn off mental stress. You can call a therapist and try to work it out in talk; you can arrange a meeting with a friend as

Dialogue #3

W: So you wouldn't blame yourself for contracting cancer — I thought I'd die anyway? Is that the message?
C: You said that, not me.
W: What then?
C: The conditions were ripe.
W: And this is what you wanted me to understand?
C: You're being obtuse. And yet, in part it's useful for you to see that the conditions were ripe. We're always here, dormant cells, if you will, waiting
W: Crap.
C: As you will. for your soul to be in distress, in trauma, that when we can invade.

← ... punish me — for something I'd done wrong, for being a bad person, for breaking ...

understanding and compassionate as my friend R, and hope to ease out of your depression on the strength of his grace and goodness. Keeping handy a video that sets you rolling on the floor with laughter may be of assistance: I stockpile copies of Eddie Murphy and Robin Williams videos at the ready. Sometimes that works; on other occasions it does not. I wish rising above depression were as easy as popping a video into the machine. You can avoid ingesting tranquilizers and other drugs that combine with the chemicals in your body to trigger depression. You can go on one of the anti-depressant drugs. You can retreat to a favourite place and try writing yourself out of the depression—by venting in an extended monologue, or by what may be called "dialoguing with your depression." Like most things that befall us, depressions pass with time; later, tomorrow, or the next day, the blackness in your soul will lift. You will come out on the other side. At the very least you can hang on to that.

-Listen: to die with meaning, see, that's what it's all about.

-Blah, blah. You're a great bore these days, dear boy.

-Here's what I mean: the man who is struck down in the street by a car, his death lacks meaning, right? Because it is sudden and pointless, such a death cheats our need for a finale. Such an event, such a passing does not bring a life to a close, it merely sees it shut down. Shut down brutally and dumbly.

-Death renders everything dumb.

-I mean inarticulate and without finish, without closure: a squirrel squashed on concrete.

-You're doing the talking.

-But if you know you're dying, if you ruminate about death, and then change things in your life, come to terms with what living means, maybe even re-invent yourself, then you give significance to your life. You bring it to a close rather than have it suddenly, randomly shut off—like water from a tap.

-That's how it is with animals. Are you saying they die without dignity?

-I'm saying human beings yearn for something greater: a parting that puts life into perspective, or at least an understanding that defines the life that led up to its ending.

-Are you saying the man who dies of a massive coronary dies unfulfilled?

-I don't know what I'm saying.

# Mortadella,
# Pecorino, Vino Aperto

*While I thought that I was learning how to live, I have been learning how to die.*

—Leonardo da Vinci

A warm October morning on a road about fifty kilometres south of Florence, Italy. It is almost ten o'clock. The sun is shining. K and I are walking south from Panzano, a hill town that looks down on a golden valley, Concho d'Oro, the locals call it. We have packs strapped to our backs. We carry water bottles and a one-and-a-half litre bottle of red wine. The dust rises up under our boots as we climb away from Panzano towards the prominence above the pines that stretch out before us and the azure sky above it. Poggio al Sodo is the name of the prominence: the southern hilltop. We study the sky; we listen to the birds; we smell oregano growing wild in the fields; we hold hands.

Two weeks earlier in Winnipeg I went for a regularly sched-uled CT scan, and a week following that, an appointment with the oncologist. During the summer, Doctor KK accepted a position at a hospital in the interior of British Columbia. So now it is Doctor WD who sees me. A middle-aged Slavic

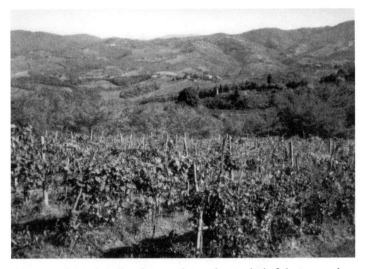

woman, she is kindly, thorough, and very helpful. At our last meeting she was immensely pleased. "You're doing so well," she told me, a smile lighting her face. She listened to my heart. She probed my intestinal area and upper groin. You know the routine: deep breath—hold it. "Mmm, mmm." She probed my liver. She tapped between my shoulder blades with the ends of her fingers. "Well, good news," she told me when I'd pulled my shirt on and was sitting opposite, "one tumour has disappeared."

"Really?"

"There was a lesion on a duct between your liver and your bowel. According to the radiologist's report, it's gone."

"Good Lord. Gone?"

"The other tumours—in the liver—are stable."

"No growth?"

"More than that. The radiologists cannot get a good read on the lesion in the terminal ileum. If they did not know it was supposed to be there, they could not see it. I'm so pleased. It must be the interferon."

"Maybe a residual effect of the I131 treatment."

"Or that. Yes." Doctor WD flipped through my thickening file. "Chromogranin at 42," she reported. At the high point two years earlier, when I'd gone off interferon in preparation for the 1131 treatment, it had hit 326. Over the intervening period it had fallen and stayed down. The past six samples were in the 20-50 range. "Very good," she said, beaming again, "these are very good results. So how are you feeling?"

Up is a feeling that every victim of cancer experiences differently. Up is a charge in the legs; up is a lightness in the chest cavity; up is turning on the stereo and belting out "The Pearl Fisher's Song" by Bizet. Up is waking at 7:30 with a clear head and red blood pounding in your veins, and after sex, making boiled eggs on toasted banana bread for breakfast before taking the off-road cycle path along the river with K on the way to her office downtown. You stretch out on the grass at the forks of the rivers and study the blue sky, smelling the water and listening to the buzz of distant traffic. You return home after twenty kilometres of vigorous aerobic activity and you shower and then you set to work sanding the cedar deck. You feel the sun on your neck and smell the lemon balm in the herb garden and you laugh aloud.

What could be better? Here is another remarkable—nay, wonderful—thing about being human that I've discovered since having cancer: no matter how bad things get, we revel in the brief moments of reprieve that come along afterwards. You remember what it was like to be a child? You may have been wounded by some event—a toy was taken away by an older sibling, say—but then in the next moment here comes Mommy with an ice-cream cone. Yippee! The moment of pain passes, replaced by joy and exhilaration. These intense feelings never really leave us, though they do become buried under the morass of adult cares, concerns, and anxieties that we all gradually take on our shoulders as we take up jobs and mortgages and so on. But you can re-open yourself to them, so that a walk on a Sunday afternoon, or the baking of gateau for your family, or crushing sage between your fingers and holding it to your nose, or sanding the cedar deck on a sunny summer afternoon become occasions of joy and celebration, become moments of genuine human ecstasy. No matter how down we may be on Monday, there is still the prospect that Tuesday will be a better day—a good day, an excellent day.

In this mood, it's possible to indulge some unconventional thoughts. Having cancer has not been a negative experience exclusively. Dealing with the disease has forced me to reassess my life in the largest sense and, consequently, prompted greater self-knowledge. As indicated earlier, this has meant acknowledging weakness and vulnerability in myself and becoming more sympathetic to them in others. Further, I have had to come to grips with my public persona and to modify the face that I present to the world. Then, too, recognizing the finiteness of time has brought into clear focus the things I truly value and the goals I wish to achieve in my lifespan. In addition, there have been unanticipated, residual side benefits. One of these concerns my threshold of anxiety. Discovering I had cancer proved to be an enormous shock, one that I would not wish on anyone. And yet, having endured that shock, having recovered from the dread of knowing that death is near at hand, has made me rather invulnerable to other shocks: I know from subsequent experiences of loss and pain, experiences that would formerly have done profound personal damage to me, that I am emotionally stronger than I was before diagnosis, not de-sensitized, but less susceptible to being wounded. I've become less fragile, less easily upset by life's minor travails. A lot that once might have distressed me, now rolls off, like the proverbial water off a duck's back.

The road south from Panzano winds past pines. Near the prominence a beat-up and tiny car sputters by, leaving a cloud of white dust in its wake. Farther along we stop at a clearing to drink water and take in the landscape. This is Poggio del Pino: tall pines, thick green grass, flies buzzing about. The air carries a scent. "Not pine," K says; maybe rosemary. We look about: a hedge of rosemary is growing behind us, three feet high and a couple of hundred feet in length. We drink a little red wine, then some more water, and then resume our walk. We come to an abandoned building, once a wine press, perhaps, more recently a home. There are curtains hanging askew on the windows. A grape arbour grows over the rear door. Sweet, lush, large, bluish grapes—Sangiovese? This is Casa del Sodo. We poke about for a while, ascertaining that no one lives at Casa del Sodo. We drink water; we eat several bunches of grapes and pluck several more, which we devour as we walk east towards the town of Lamole, our lips turning purple as we spit seeds onto the gravel at our feet.

Sun on the skin, dust in the nostrils, scent of rosemary.

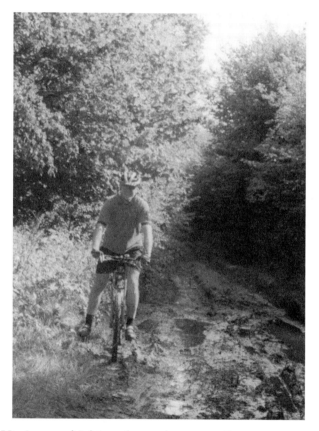

Up is not thinking about aberrant cells or CT scans or Chromogranin A. Up is a place in the mind far removed from embolization and radioactive isotopes. As we descend the gravel road to Lamole we sing "Jesus Is on the Main Line" by Ry Cooder, and then "Waltzing Mathilda" makes an appearance before we enter the town of Lamole, where heavy, blue grapes grow in vineyards along the road. Up is stopping for photos of the grapes and then of a deeply tanned man driving a tractor with a small tin wagon attached behind; he's hauling the harvested grapes to a golden stone building just down the road. At the *pieve* in the town centre we slip out of our backpacks and open the parcels of food we bought at the *alimentari* in Panzano: pecorino fresco, olives, panne, mortadella. Up is sipping red wine and dropping bread crumbs down the front of your shirt while looking across the valley toward the prominence we just came from, the green of pines, the blue of sky, the mixed pungencies of the *vendemmia*. Having a disease and feeling ill inhabit another country. Up is living in the moment, enjoying each particle of happiness that falls to us. Up is trekking through the Monti del Chianti, twenty kilometres a day up and down dusty hills in the heat; is having the courage to take on something that could be stressful, painful, or both, but more likely will be joyful and good for the soul. Seizing the day.

K sighs. She is a long way from the stress of her legal practice. I have not had a gut ache since we arrived in Italy, more than a week ago. I sleep through the night. We drink a litre and a half of wine with lunch and another litre or so with our supper. There is no such thing as liver failure or flushing or cancer. We do not remember the last time we uttered the dismal phrase "carcinoid syndrome."

-J is dead, dear boy.

-You bastards.

-See, his obit in your precious little carcinoid journal.

-He edited that publication. He was painstaking and generous in distributing it. He believed it was important to put information into the hands of carcinoid patients. To provide scientific fact and to give hope.

-Now he's dead. Your eighteen-year survivor, your paragon, your ray of hope. You secretly modelled yourself on him, right? So what message do you take from this obituary, this notice of his death?

-You utter bastards.

-We win, see.

-You gloat. But—

-But what? What is there to say in the face of Death?

-You ...we ...

-See, see!

# Rollercoaster

*Life is a tragedy when seen in close-up, but a comedy in long-shot.*

—Charlie Chaplin

Having cancer is a rollercoaster ride: one day up; the next day down. First, on top of the world; then the plunge to the bottom. Whee! There's a certain element of the carnival in the procedure, especially as *carne-val* refers to the weaknesses of the human flesh. Having cancer whips you from the dizzying heights of exhilaration to the pit of gloom. Whee! Only having cancer does not feel like *whee*; it feels like *whoa*.

The carnival is a place where ordinary expectations and responses do not apply. When we visit the fair and take a ride on the rollercoaster, we freely invite a kind of giddy mayhem into our lives. We submit ourselves to the titillation of apprehended disaster—embracing a version of calamity in order to experience hair-raising sensations. We know that accidents occur on these wild rides from time to time, but mostly we trust that our fairground flirtations with catastrophe will amount to no more than a brief but hair-raising thrill. To a minor—but exhilarating—degree our lives will be out of control; but only to a minor degree, and only for a fleeting time.

Having cancer, or being subject to any serious disease or ailment, means being permanently out of control; means being subject to many shocks, to being continuously vulnerable, and never in charge. Think of it this way. If you fall and twist your ankle, you know the steps back to recovery because they conform to a predictable schedule: you visit the sports doctor; you have the X-rays; you take the prescribed medications; you do the physiotherapy; you gingerly manoeuvre about on your feet for a while. If you apply yourself to the healing with conviction, your injury will recover and you will return to normal within some weeks. Good as new. The damage is—given certain limits—within your control. Many illnesses work this way: most accidental injuries and a large percentage of afflictions are self-terminating. So too are dependencies. Even the alcoholic can rise one day and say, "That's enough. I'm going to quit." And with the right measure of determination, with dedicated support, and with lots of fallback, the alcoholic can reverse his terrible predicament. In a very important way, the alcoholic has mastery over his condition and can regain control of his life.

Not so with cancer. Contracting cancer, being a victim of disease, means loss of control. Now the carnival ride is out of one's hands. Other forces—malign, mysterious, and awesome forces—are directing the journey. Life no longer feels like an adventure, but rather a perilous plunge into the dark unknown with deranged demons at the controls, while your heart hammers hard and sweat starts from your brow. Vertigo. Whoa!

In one sense you become an open wound of emotions, subject to instant reversals of feeling. Every newspaper article extolling some recent development in labs with rats raises your hopes. Every suggestion that things may not be going well in your body cuts like a knife. For example. Shortly after discovering that you have cancer, you are talking to a former colleague and friend. JH cares about you; he is sympathetic to your fragile emotions; he wants to know about your condition. This is several weeks after you have been diagnosed, when the dramatic first shock wave of having cancer has passed. You have read some literature; you have spoken with the physicians; you think you understand the "curve" of the disease and what lies in store for you. You have reached a kind of emotional plateau. You think you are no longer subject to the shock of *cancer*. So you begin having visitors over for tea and subdued chats in the sitting room: everyone wants to know how you are doing; it's only fair for you to let them see.

JH is a slight and nervous man in his early forties. As he talks he runs one hand through his sandy hair. He is agitated but I assure him I'm all right. We sit in leather chairs opposite each other. I say a few things about the way I came to be diagnosed, and then add, "There are tumours in the liver." We are relaxing with our cups of tea. JH looks at me over the rim of his cup, brown eyes widening. "Oh my," he says, running his hand through his hair several times, "the liver, that's bad now, isn't it?" And on these otherwise innocuous words, down I plunge. My heart races. Does JH know something I do not? Have the physicians hidden something from me? Have I misunderstood the articles in the journals? Did Doctor KO give me false hope? Will I die soon? Have I been building castles in the air? My stomach tightens, the first indicator of stress. Sweating, I'm on the precipitous fall from a giddy height. Emotional vertigo. If only JH would leave so I could regain emotional equilibrium and go on dealing with the cancer alone—free from the unthinking wounds of friends, their words that spin me out of control.

It may take months or years before you lose this hyper sensitivity to the issue of *cancer*. Most of the time you avoid the word altogether: it reverberates with too many painful associations. You notice that your friends and relatives do the same, telling you only that celebrity X or acquaintance Y has passed away. Intuitively everyone grasps how subject you have become to the reckless rollercoaster ride.

In the western world we put a lot of store on being in control. We like to feel that we make the important decisions in our lives—our careers, where and how we live, our sexual partners, the number of children we raise, and so on. A lot of emphasis is put on independence and self-activation, buzz words that remind us that being in charge of one's own life is not only desirable but important. Further, we admire people who exhibit self-control: movie actors who portray heroes with nerves of steel and determination knit on their brows are constantly lionized. Television commercials flogging everything from automobiles to women's sanitary products advise us to take control. Sports figures exhort us to Be The Man. The message is that we empower ourselves through mastery of life. We sense that when we lose control our lives are less ours, less integrated, less worthy than when we exercise control.

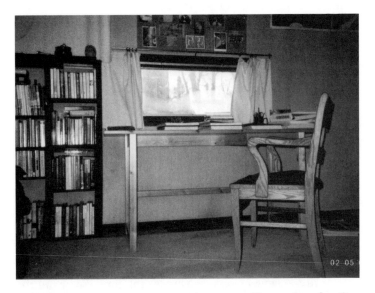

Having cancer means accepting an unlike and unfamiliar set of parameters for our lives, means submitting ourselves to the whims of microscopic demons inside our bodies. This relinquishing of control can be extremely difficult for most of us to accept, an alien way of thinking, a passive attitude to our current behaviour and our future prospects that goes against our usual conviction that our future is a matter for us to determine, to structure, and to achieve. When it comes to day-to-day events, we prefer to believe that we are in charge; we do not like the idea that we have to place our faith in forces beyond our reach. We resist the insinuation that our own wishes and desires matter not; we become rancorous in the face of our frailty; we act out; we refuse to acknowledge our desperate condition. Despite a mass of evidence to the contrary, we insist on being in charge. ("It's my life," we insist to ourselves.) And yet when an oncologist announces, "Your biopsy came back positive," or you sense your body succumbing to one of the symptoms of your disease, or you wake in the night sweating or flushing or trembling uncontrollably, you feel your feverish heart flutter with the truth of your predicament, it becomes obvious that you are no longer in control. You have to accept that you are taking a journey on the emotional rollercoaster called Kancer Karnival—one tick of the clock up; the next tick down.

-Dear boy, what's all the ruckus? Wine, toasts, hullabaloo in the kitchen?

-Good news—for me.

-Don't gloat, it's unbecoming.

-The results of my latest scan, see. The tumour in the terminal ileum gone.

-Can't be seen on scan, you mean. That's a different thing.

-You cannot bring me down. Primary tumour gone. But that's not all. Tumours in the liver smaller than before. Shrinkage. Receding. The battle is being won.

-Temporary. An illusion.

-But it's good news, that's the point. I'm up. The interferon is working, the doctors say.

-It's only temporary. Cancer finds a way to win out. Mutating cells, dear boy, mutate in all kinds of ways and get around the interferon. Eventually. Kill you in the end.

-You cannot bring me down. Not today. The improvement is slow, the doctors say. But it is progress.

-Cancer mutates into hundreds—thousands—of new forms, into classes the interferon cannot keep up to, much less combat. That's why AIDS will never be defeated; there are too many fresh aberrations for the drugs to overcome. It's the same with cancer. Aberrant cells find a way around the interferon. Eventually.

-Carping, *dear boy*. You cannot bring me down. Not today.

# Scent of Pine

*In my room the world is beyond my understanding;*
*but when I walk I see that it consists of three or four*
*hills and a cloud.*

—Wallace Stevens

Facing death is not easy. Shakespeare reminds us of how difficult it is when he has Hamlet ruminate on the "sleep of death," and concludes that "conscience doth make cowards of us all." I do not know if I am either more knowledgeable about death or wiser in facing it for having contracted cancer and, consequently, looked death in the face. I do know that whatever I now think is fired with the flame of experience and felt along the bone in a way that was not true before. In other words, as a college student, in common with millions of other such students, I came to understand from wide reading in the classic texts what mankind has thought about death over the span of human history; but it is only since contracting cancer that I have sensed what it is like to feel the cold hand of Death gripping my shoulder.

So I make so bold as to share a few thoughts I've had since being diagnosed.

We know that we are going to die; we know that some day we will no longer walk this enchanting and delightful earth. Our bodies will corrupt in the earth, our loved ones will go forward into time without us at their sides. People will rise in the morning, make coffee, eat toast, plan the kitchen renovation, but we will not be there to see their smiles, hear their laughter, smell their hair. The poet Wordsworth said it this way: life's diurnal course will go on, but we will not be here to enjoy the round. These can be upsetting and depressing thoughts. They are the sometimes terrifying facts that we do possess about death. What to do, what to think in the face of them?

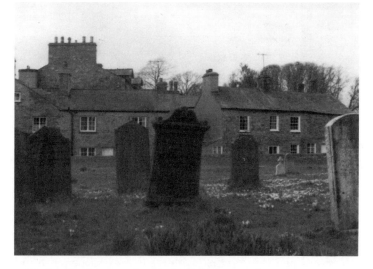

Dying is change, the biggest change we have to encounter in this life. Most of us do not like change; most of us resist it in whatever form it presents itself. Yet change is one of the ever-present realities of this life: we grow; we grow up; we become adults with our own children; we lose hair; we gain weight; we move from this place to that, from this job to that; we grow old. And so on. Accepting change is accepting the process that is life; embracing change is acknowledging that we are born, we procreate, we die. You need look no farther than the book of Ecclesiastes to know that only by accepting change can we truly embrace life. The momentous change that we call dying is the end-point of a process that began with our birth and may not conclude with the moment we cease to breathe and give off electrical energy on this earth. There may be something after death. We do not know about that. We do know that everyone dies and that we must, however unwillingly, face the reality of the weighty change we call death.

There are, of course, many ways of dealing with the knowledge that you are dying. One is denial, looking away from the reality of death, refusing to acknowledge and accept that knowledge. Though not recommended by most health-care workers and therapists, the effectiveness of this strategy is not to be dismissed. Animals are not conscious of death, of the fact that they are dying. As far as we know, they simply live and then die, unaware that death awaits them, and content, it seems, with moving through this earthly experience. Their blissful ignorance is perhaps to be envied. But we humans are not in their happy position; we have consciousness, and early in our life we become aware that everyone dies, that we ourselves will die, especially once we contract certain illnesses. So it's a terrible curse as well as a blessing, our human consciousness. Still, some of us can (through willpower) turn away from this knowledge and live out our days, refusing to acknowledge our impending demise. This may, in one sense, be a very healthy way to deal with death. There is some evidence, some physicians and researchers suggest, to support the usefulness of denial in the treatment of terminal illness. Bernie Siegel, for instance, while not recommending denial as a course of action, reports the case of a busy middle-aged gardener with a stomach cancer who lived for many years, telling Siegel whenever he visited him—to once again postpone surgery—"I just can't take time from my gardening to have cancer." So, denial.

A more common course of response to the frightening prospect of death is to turn to religion. Churches, synagogues, mosques, and other like institutions offer a number of valuable constructs in the face of death. A collective of like-minded believers, a pattern of ritual established over time, and a deity to turn to in periods of crisis are only the three most obvious of these. All offer support, encouragement, and a rationale for life's most bewildering reality, its termination. Indeed, it is this last virtue, the rationale, that is often most important to victims of terminal illness. Religion proffers to believers a complete world view, including an explanation of the origins of existence, and the meaning of time on the earth. It answers the questions *why do we die?* and *where are we going to after this existence?* A great many victims of cancer turn to religion for these explanations and find them both comforting and strengthening. Though I have no statistics at hand to ratify the claim, I would hazard the guess that almost everyone who contracts cancer becomes, as a result, a more spiritual person than they were previously. At the very least, most victims of cancer become kinder people than they were before. You could say there's a kind of cosmic compensation at work in our beings when we develop a terminal illness: the fragility of our body is counter-balanced by the resiliency of our spirit.

I have always been fascinated by the stoical position. You will recall, perhaps, that this is where Shakespeare himself ends up, having Hamlet say of death, "If it be now, 'tis not to come; if it be not to come, it will be now; if it be not now, yet it will come." Rather than being enraged or depressed by this conundrum, Hamlet seems positively relieved by it, concluding, "The readiness is all." Being prepared to leave this wonderful existence, this blessing we call life. In short, our readiness to accept dying matters more than when or how we die. Would that we could learn to embrace this attitude!

The fundamental issue here, I believe, is trust. By that I mean that as victims of a terminal illness we must put ourselves in the hands of something (God?), trusting our future to forces outside our own control. We're not used to that; we seek to control, to be in charge. Further, we have learned in our private lives and our careers to find resolution to problems, to seek closure. But when we develop a cancer we come to realize that we are not in control and that the issue with our diseases may never be resolved the way we want it to be. Even if we are "cured" (no cancer for five years), it may rebound. And most of us are not so fortunate as to be cured: we go on with our days, enduring the agony of pain, the indignity of hospitals, the debilitation of suffering, the confusions of not knowing what is going to happen next. So we must trust ourselves to live without resolution, without closure. We must arrive at the point where trust takes over, becomes our way of life, and where we take each day for what it is and embrace it.

Taking that step to trust means humbling the self, acknowledging that we do not and cannot control our own fate. In some circles the act of humbling the self is called "going down into the ashes." The phrase reminds us that humility is a matter of giving up pride in the most basic of ways, of exposing oneself before others in the way that certain prophets do in spiritual texts. Stripping the self naked; prostrating oneself on the humble terra firma. These are difficult acts, especially for middle-aged men who have enjoyed success, achievement, and status, who are accustomed to looking down, rather than up. Self-effacement is not one of the

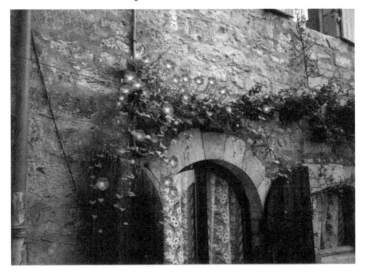

requirements of being a CEO or earning the six-figure salary. So such gestures are almost as forbidding to perform as they are necessary for true healing to occur.

My mother, eighty-two, frail of heart and the last surviving member on both sides of my lineage (some twenty-six uncles and aunts of my own having died), says to me, "I close my eyes every night in bed not knowing whether I'm going to wake up in the morning. So I'm grateful for each day when I do re-awake and rediscover I'm still here." This, I suppose, is the message behind living life: counting each day as a gift and treating each experience as a blessing. The ancients had a phrase for this: *carpe diem*, seize the day. They knew that life was short— much shorter than in our time—and that the only real response to the prospect of death was to live whatever time they had been granted to the fullest extent possible. Or so, at least, they wrote. I have found it is not easy to live up to the exhilarating sentiment behind *carpe diem;* to honour each sunrise, to cherish each apple, to wax poetic about each child's achievement; much less applaud every television commercial and exclaim over the rainy days. We are creatures of habit, we humans, and among our habits are grumbling over faults in others and sighing over dreary days. It's a challenge to try to transform such negative habits, to greet each day with enthusiasm and a sprightly step. Being of sanguine temperament helps. Being surrounded by upbeat friends and family does too. On days when I feel as low as the soles of my shoes, I can be instantly energized, for instance, by overhearing my son quietly whistling to himself as he plays with his Lego on the carpet of the family room. Trying to sing every day helps. Doing things for friends and family. It's not only fun but life-enhancing to prepare each evening meal with the care and enthusiasm we usually reserve for the big dinners on festive occasions. Greeting a neighbour over the backyard fence. Noting the flora and fauna encountered on a walk can bring a smile to the lips and a skip to the beleaguered heart. And so on. It's all we have. It's what makes being here rich and exciting.

There's also what might be referred to as the "Zen of small

tasks," taking pride in doing the best job possible of every chore around the house: sweeping the floors, for instance. I make a point of whistling as I clean the toilets. Tasks that once irritated me—collecting up the fall leaves—can be a positive delight. As can going for a walk and looking up at the clouds and hills. It's been somewhat painful to come to the following recognition, but it's a crucial one: I'm not going anywhere, I now realize, and no one is; the world is not waiting on us to do something important. Nothing we will ever do is, ultimately, important. Would that I had learned this lesson earlier—would that some of my friends and relatives could learn it yet. We're not going anywhere but to the grave, so why do we tie ourselves up in knots over deadlines and schedules and ascending the career ladder? Well, we know the answer, sad as it is: ambition, fear, arrogance, anxiety, the whole stew of human frailties.

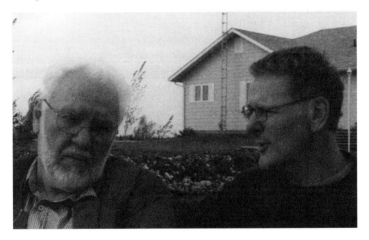

In the end, we hope to learn from all life's happenings, and the experience of having a terminal illness, cancer included, is one of these. In addition, we hope to transform the giant negative that is disease into something positive, living with it, and living through it, re-inventing ourselves each day to face the new realities that change brings, so that our days will not only be a pleasure to ourselves, but also to those we have been blessed to find around us.

-I'm saying that death is a state, an unhappy state, true, but I'm also saying that dying is one of life's processes, like growing taller.

-Or shorter.

-Yes, as we grow older and die out of life we become shorter. We diminish. We spend many years coming to the point where we accept that; where we accept that that is a condition of our condition.

-More philosophy—eastern, no?

-I agree with the poet who said dying is a process in the same way living is a process.

-This fancy talk comes to little more than denial; it will not get you out of it, though. It will not save you from death.

-Still you insist on scaring me with death?

-You are not afraid of death?

-Of course. I do not want to *not* be here. Here is good. I was listening to Puccini last evening; I was sipping a mossy Scotch. On the couch beside me sat my beautiful wife; my painfully wonderful son played on the floor. Here, this earth, this set of loves is great. We would all like to live forever, and we feel a sharp pain in the heart, an insult to our beings to sense that some day this precious "I" we call our human selves will not be here. Taking death in, really taking it in brings on a gasp of self-pity, the kind of desolation we feel as teenagers but rarely as adults. I do not want to die. But I see now that dying is not a failure. So you can no longer throw it up at me that way. You cannot terrify me with this word: Death.

-Death is reality.

-It is one reality, and only in this sense: that we all die. But far more important is how we die. If we can die out of life, then ...

-"Die out of life"?

-Recognizing that life and death are phases in a process means accepting change, and then trusting in larger forces to guide that change, so that ultimately we trust our lives to something greater than ourselves and accept change, even if it is not positive change.

-Process? Your life is not so much cheese.

-But fear of death is the fear of change, the fear of process.

-You are not afraid of change?

-Life is change: we come and we go—and in a blink of the universe's eye. Life is a stream rushing down a hill—nothing remains the same for long in a stream rushing down a hill.

-You sound like a professor. Worse, a professor with a smattering of Buddhism or whatever. *Process, change, significance.* Really!

-Yes. It's a bit of a mouthful and can sound preachy, I admit, but this is what we come to know on this earth: embrace change and you embrace life.

-And death?

-Yes—accept our passing as we accept our being here, our living, our joys and our frustrations. If we can see our little circumscribed existence as a blessing, a gift of the cosmos, if we can die out of life, then we can truly live. Accept change as the one constant of life and you at once embrace the process of dying and the wonder of living.

# Epilogue

*Sickness enlarges the dimensions of a man's self to himself.*

—Charles Lamb

In writing the preceding pages I may have communicated the impression that I have dealt with cancer systematically and successfully, a victory story. But that is a false lead. I have not in any real sense beaten cancer. I might never, given the type of cancer I have and the general prognosis for this variety— which is that death follows twelve to eighteen years after inception of the disease. Still, I was conscious in the writing— and more conscious in the reading of what I have written— that I had assumed (perhaps *affected* is more accurate) the pose of the all-knowing schoolmaster offering counsel and advice to the untutored. I tried not to have this tone take over my ruminations; but I fear I may not have succeeded as fully as I wished.

Once you have been diagnosed, dealing with cancer day-to-day is an up-and-down experience. Mondays, Wednesdays, and Fridays you feel pretty good about yourself; the other days, not. It's more than an on-and-off daily trial; as I indicated in one chapter, it's a rollercoaster—physical, emotional, intellectual. It sweeps you along; it controls you. It wears you out—and wears you down. Much of the time you feel helpless; even though when you come to write about what's happened—and continues to happen—you adopt the tone of someone who's in charge. The writing itself is partly responsible for this effect: writing is a product of the reflection and the surmise that come with contemplation after the event, whereas the disease is a matter of immediate reactions and suffering. (I have tried to capture something of the latter in the dialogues inserted as *entre actes* between chapters.)

So I wanted to make clear that whatever impression my preachy tone may have created, I am daily living with this disease—and struggling with it and my own responses to it. Some days I'm down; some up. It's a lot like a normal life, only more compressed and more exaggerated. Everything seems urgent, intense. Much of the time I feel as you feel when you're undergoing one of life's critical experiences: falling in love, grieving a death, contemplating a career change, having a baby, and so on: nervous energy with nowhere to go, heart palpitations. Subject, that is, to emotions beyond my control, and aware that the door of the kitchen cupboard opens onto the lane of the dead.

I've been conscious throughout the writing, too, of a degree of phoniness in my position as a cancer patient. Carcinoid syndrome is a gentle cancer. Laugh here. Its symptoms are mild things such as flushing, fever, diarrhea, and shortness of breath. You are not—at least not often—stricken with sharp pains, or overpowering nausea, or subject to wrenching illness—vomiting and the like. Patients of carcinoid cancer do not spend a lot of time attached to IV machines; they do not suffer dramatic weight fluctuations, or spectacular loss of hair. Up to the end, they are not bed-ridden. We do not have giant tumours in our bodies that make us unsightly. Do I need to go on? So there's something a little askew in a person suffering this particular cancer taking it on himself to write about having cancer.

It is, though, a terminal cancer: people who contract carcinoid cancer are not cured. Current treatments can hold it off, but that is the best we can hope for. No inspiring Lance Armstrong triumph over cancer for carcinoid patients. After a number of years the tumours in our livers or lungs grow to the point where they disable our healthy organs; the chemicals eat away at other tissue—many die of failure of the right side of the heart. Painfully and at length. All that aside, it's been useful to me to think about this disease, and, hence, I've thought it might be useful for others to read about this one journey. In reflecting on what's happened to me and how I've reacted to it, I've come to understand myself better. That's an achievement I'm happy to report. I've also learned a lot of things from others; they deserve a place here, too. *Yay* to you all. To patients of carcinoid cancer and other cancers I finally say this: hang in there; it's not that bad.

# Afterword:
# Speaking the "c" Word

*It is foolish to tear one's hair in grief, as though sorrow would be made less by baldness.*

—Cicero

Among the issues of immediate importance that face the recently diagnosed cancer patient, there is one that receives less attention than it should: whether to reveal that one has contracted the disease; and how to tell people about the affliction without upsetting others or oneself.

In the not-so-distant past cancer was regarded as a death sentence. In the fifties and sixties people who had cancer were usually in the final phases of their lives: diagnostic techniques were nowhere near as sophisticated as they are at present—nor were the treatments and drugs available to counter the disease that are available today to victims of cancer. To learn that someone had cancer meant that you should prepare for their imminent demise. That can still be true today. Many cancers are not easily detectable until they are far advanced in our bodies; others are of the virulent, "racing," variety: within weeks or months of diagnosis, patients succumb. So over time we have become—quite rightly—very wary of the word "cancer": it spells the end of someone's life, and of our relationship with them. We resist the distress of acknowledging someone else's suffering.

How, then, to tell people, especially those close to us, that we have cancer?

My own mother, who grew up with six siblings who lived to adulthood, not to mention the family of my father, her in-laws, also a set of seven adult siblings, has witnessed many deaths from cancer. Her mother-in-law succumbed to an intestinal variety; two of her sisters died of leukemia; one of her brothers of lung cancer. Following my diagnosis, I spoke to my sisters, as noted in an earlier chapter. When we had dealt with our various feelings, our anxieties focussed on our mother, who was then seventy-four years of age, and with a frail heart. We were in a quandary about telling her; we were not sure what to do. There's an inevitable panic that strikes us when we learn someone close has cancer: we feared for *her* health. In addition, we were uncertain how the disease would develop, how much time I had before my condition became critical—or I died. My sisters and I waited four or five months, feeling guilty all the time that we had not revealed my condition to our mother. Then when the course of my illness became more clear to us, and when I felt more balanced about the future, my sisters and I visited my mother. It was on a Tuesday evening, an oddity for all three of her busy children (especially without their children) to drop by on our mother. After we'd chatted for a few minutes, I drew a deep breath and plunged in. My mother's face turned ashen; her lower lip trembled. "Cancer," she said, "oh no." Tears, inability to speak, fierce trembling. My sisters had wisely sat one on each side of her on the divan; they were able to embrace her and comfort her. And in a while she took possession of herself again. My older sister made tea; my younger sister went over the prognosis again, telling our mother that carcinoid syndrome is a slow-moving variety of cancer; though terminal, a patient may live with it a decade or longer. I added my own reassurances: I felt strong; I was taking up the issue with the disease; I had good care. My mother gathered herself together; she asked, "You've told me everything, you're not hiding anything?" We had not come to her with the horrifying news right away, and she was wary now that we were keeping the worst from her. She was waiting for the other shoe to drop. We reassured her as best we could. We drank our tea, and Mother wiped her tears away. We were all shaken. One of Mother's sisters had struggled bravely against leukemia over a five-year period: Mother knew that story. Her other sister had been diagnosed with leukemia on a Friday and then died on the following Monday: Mother knew that story too.

After Mother had embraced me and blown her nose for the umpteenth time, she whispered, "I'm glad your father's not alive; he couldn't have dealt with this." She's borne up pretty well since then; she asks about the CT scans; clips articles from the newspapers; buys me nutritional supplements: milk thistle, shark cartilage, and so on.

When we told my mother-in-law, her reaction was not a lot different. She was sitting in her own kitchen when K told her, "Wayne has cancer." She stood instantly, crossed the room, and embraced me. "Oh, my God, cancer," she gasped, "the worst." Her own mother had died of cancer some fifteen years earlier—following a terrible, painful struggle. One of her brothers-in-law had been coping with the disease for a decade. So, she was shaken, and our assurances that carcinoid cancer would not end my life immediately did not make an instant impression on her. She was afraid for both of us—as mothers will be—and feared for my son, A, too, as grandmothers do.

She looks at me out of the corner of her eye sometimes, when she thinks I'm not aware of it: has he lost weight, is his skin colour good, is he becoming frail? She tells K, "Wayne's doing great; he looks after himself." So on the surface, and after seven years have passed, she's coping well. But her mother died of cancer; in the years since I was diagnosed, her brother-in-law has died; she's waiting for the other shoe to drop.

So what do we do about this business of telling relatives?

The simple answer is this: tell them. They need to know; they have to internalize the information and then go about doing whatever it is they can to help. But brace yourself, too; know that *cancer* still frightens people; it shakes them to the core of their beings. Instead of receiving their immediate commiseration, you may have to comfort and reassure them. Be prepared for that reversal of roles, too. Be strong; be balanced; be forthright. Think—impossible as it can be at times—*it's just cancer.*

Telling acquaintances, people you encounter in the workplace, or on the nineteenth green, or over the backyard fence, is another matter. After a few experiences, you can predict what is going to happen: the whispered *oh, my,* the reluctant step backward, the trembling lower lip or shaking voice. Some people give you the distinct impression that this is news they would rather not have heard, not have been burdened with. You learn to gauge who can be told. Men and women differ. Women are more open to your pain and confusion; men are often more confused themselves than are women. Perhaps men are more frightened and less able to cope with this kind of stress. In any event, blabbing your news to everyone is not a wise course of action; but then neither is telling no one at all: suppressing disclosure leaves you alone, fighting the disease in silence and without the moral and emotional support that sufferers of all serious illnesses need.

At the workplace, cancer can seem, or rather can be perceived to be, a kind of failure on the part of the victim. Some people, probably again more men than women, and probably those in positions of authority more than those not in such positions, judge a victim of disease much in the same way as they regard criminals: they perceive the victim as somehow having fallen short. They blame the victim for being ill. Some employers may not want to have a cancer patient on the payroll, thinking they will erode morale, or introduce an undesirable tone in the office; some colleagues may view a cancer patient as a weak link on the team. So, rightly or wrongly, people who are diagnosed with cancer often cover up the fact, keeping the affliction and whatever pain they experience a closely guarded secret. That clandestine behaviour is unfortunate, as stressful, I conjecture, as keeping any part of one's life locked away from friends and colleagues—be it a romantic affair, or a terrifying incident, such as rape.

Each patient of a terminal illness has to deal with this issue for themselves. I have found disclosure, judiciously handled, to be a positive factor in my dealings with cancer. I told my son when he was not yet three years old, assuring him that his dad would be with him for some time to come, and reassuring him that he was in no way to blame for my condition, since children are liable to take these things on themselves. He's dealing with the issue as best he can, talking with K and me, and occasionally with his mother. Should he show signs of trauma, we will take him to a psychologist. In the meantime, he sees that I'm okay; he sees that I'm dealing with the disease as best I can. No doubt he has paid a price, emotionally, in having this knowledge thrust on him, but then would keeping the disease a secret have led to even greater emotional damage, and to distance between us? I think so.

In a larger context, I've mentioned in the preceding pages that I play on sports teams. Up to the time of diagnosis, I played hockey three times a week, with two different sets of enthusiasts. At first I did not tell my locker mates. I played alongside my nephew, twenty years my junior, on a competitive team. For some months we told no one else—I had the feeling SW was a little ashamed of my condition—but then one day I had to explain my absence during an earlier game, and I quietly revealed my condition to the fellows sitting nearby. Followed the predictable silence. What is there to say? But in the subsequent months no one made an issue of the disclosure one way or the other. Perhaps some teammates felt I had crossed a line by making a personal predicament public. If they did, I did not hear about their restiveness. What I did hear was quiet support from almost every teammate, but one at a time and in private moments—inquiries into my state of health, reserved but sincere pats on the shoulder, offers to help. When I recently divulged my condition to a locker mate who had inquired about this book, he said, "I'm sorry to hear that—but don't expect me to go easy on you out there because of it." I hadn't, and he knew it, of course. Disclosure does not mean asking for pity, merely acknowledging a fact.

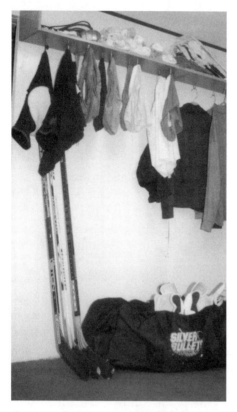

If you trust others with your vulnerability, I've discovered, they'll stand by you—and respect you, to boot. We're living in an age when even strong silent types, like teammates in a locker room, are open to sharing each part of your life and are sincere about their support for your struggle. After all, it's a fairly well-known fact that about half of the male population will contract some form, some degree, of cancer in their lifetimes—as it is also widely understood that about twenty per cent of women will experience a brush with breast cancer. There is hardly anything secretive about the disease any more—much less shameful. Celebrities such as Lance Armstrong endorse fund-raising projects; legendary figures like Tom Watts publicly discuss their recovery on video bites. Talk radio; books such as this one. In a world that every week witnesses another sports hero weeping openly on television about minor misdemeanours or blubbering farewells to the game, quietly revealing a diagnosis seems very unlikely to erode one's manhood or womanhood.

In brief, I have experienced the profound decency of acquaintances and their heartfelt sympathy; so I feel good about having told people about my condition, and I encourage others to broach the subject of *cancer* as thoroughly as they feel able.